**Praise for Juliet Sullivan's** *The Gallstone-friendly Diet..*

*'The Gallstone-friendly Diet* is an amusing and informative journey.'
James Hopkins FRCS, Metabolic and Bariatric Surgeon, Bristol, UK

'An excellent and amusing book with all the facts you need.'
Veronica McQuade, UK

'Juliet makes you feel as though you are getting advice from a close friend. Unlike typical self-help books, this one will have you laughing, engaged… and making delicious gallbladder-friendly food!'
Donna Moore, Canada

'Juliet Sullivan recounts her personal story in a very honest way. She takes you through her surgery and out the other side. Unfortunately for her, she spent five months suffering from her gallstones before having her gallbladder removed. Fortunately for us, as a result of this wait she has produced a wonderful selection of recipes that are less likely to initiate pain than are standard meals. This is a truly helpful read, but if you've got gallstones, get an operation soon!'
Giles J Toogood, Professor of Hepatobiliary Surgery
University of Leeds, Leeds, UK

'I love Juliet's humour and wit. As I am dealing with gallbladder issues, this book is perfect timing as I have had no idea what to expect. I have information now to help me understand what I am dealing with. Thank you!'
Lorelei, Texas, USA

'Juliet Sullivan does a brilliant job of enlightening her audience with the facts that are necessary for understanding gallstones. Additionally, the recipes contained in this book serve as a really useful guide for anyone struggling with the dietary issues associated with gallstones. Considering that gallstones are a serious illness, Juliet Sullivan uses her humour to address the elements of unease and fear that can be associated with a diagnosis, and to assist those who struggle in navigating the lifestyle changes that will be needed. All in all, I give this book a 5/5. Fantastic job!'
Nicole Irvine, Canada

*For my mother, Margaret, and father, Ron. Though imperfect, complicated and eccentric, they are of course the reason for me – and by extension my two amazing children – being here. They would be delighted to know they received a dedication in this book, despite its contents.*

# What becomes of the broken-hearted

Broken-heart syndrome
(aka takotsubo cardiomyopathy),
my mother's suicide and other stories

## Juliet Sullivan

With a Foreword by Caron Curragh

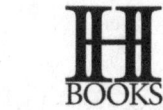

Hammersmith Health Books
London, UK

This first edition is published by Hammersmith Health Books – an imprint of Hammersmith Books Limited
4/4A Bloomsbury Square, London WC1A 2RP, UK
www.hammersmithbooks.co.uk

© 2025, Juliet Sullivan

The right of Juliet Sullivan has been asserted by her in accordance with the Copyright, Designs and Patents Act 1988.

All rights reserved. No part of this publication may be reproduced, stored in any retrieval system or transmitted in any form or by any means, electronic, mechanical, photocopying, recording or otherwise, without the prior permission of the publishers and copyright holders.

The information contained in this book is for educational purposes only. It is the result of the study and the experience of the author. Whilst the information and advice offered are believed to be true and accurate at the time of going to press, neither the author nor the publisher can accept any legal responsibility or liability for any errors or omissions that may have been made or for any adverse effects which may occur as a result of following the recommendations given herein. Always consult a qualified medical practitioner if you have any concerns regarding your health.

British Library Cataloguing in Publication Data: A CIP record of this book is available from the British Library.

Print ISBN 978-1-78161-262-0
Ebook ISBN 978-1-78161-263-7

Commissioning editor: Georgina Bentliff
Designed and typeset by: Julie Bennett of Bespoke Publishing Ltd
Cover design by: Madeline Meckiffe
Cover photograph: © jingpixar/RawPixel
Index: Jan Ross
Production: Angela Young
Printed and bound by: TJ Books Ltd, Cornwall, UK

# Contents

**Foreword by Caron Curran**    vii
**Acknowledgements**    xi
**Note from the Author**    xiii

**Part I: Home is where the (broken) heart is**    1
Introduction    3
1. Before the heartbreak    5
2. Digging deep: tales from a troubled childhood    13
3. A silent witness to mental illness    23
4. Octopus: our safe word    29
5. My mother's suicide    35
6. One funeral and a wedding    39
7. Back to reality    47
8. Be still my broken heart    51
9. Friday the 13th    57
10. A life without stress    65
11. In the aftermath    71

**Part II: Understanding the octopus pot syndrome**    77
12. The fun stuff    79
13. Expert opinions on takotsubo    93
14. Stories of takotsubo    115

**Part III: Looking after your heart health**    **169**
15. Heart-healthy recipes    171
16. About suicide    213

**References**    **219**
**Resources**    **221**
**Index**    **225**

# Foreword

'We know there's still something wrong with your heart; we're not quite sure what, but at your age you will learn to live with it.' These were the parting words of the doctor who discharged me from hospital in October 2013 after I had had a nearly fatal, unusual type of heart failure known as takotsubo syndrome (TTS).

The causation of the attack that almost ended my life had in all probability begun four weeks earlier, when I was involved in a road traffic accident and had been taken to hospital. There, I was told that the mid-back, breastbone and slight chest pain I was experiencing were probably due to the seat belt snapping across my chest after the impact of the other car.

Fast-forward four weeks, and still feeling unwell, I had a disagreement with a neighbour who had been blocking our driveway for four days with piles of bricks and sand. My polite request for them to move this onto their land led to a strong retort. Getting nowhere, I went indoors. I quietly closed my front door, but my heart did the complete opposite; it went 'boom!'

Paramedics were called and I was taken to hospital. After being triaged, I was told I needed to see a doctor, only to sit in A&E (Emergency) for around eight hours. My whole body was shaking; I was turning blue and trying to focus on my breathing. At 11:00 pm, I was eventually seen, had various cardiac diagnostics performed and was admitted onto a ward.

When my blood results finally came through, panic ensued. I was told that there was something seriously wrong with my heart and I needed to be moved to a different hospital. Following an angiogram at the second hospital, I was finally diagnosed with a severe attack of a particular type of heart failure, namely takotsubo.

After a four-day stay in the first hospital, I heard the words from the doctor I mentioned in my introduction: 'At your age you will learn to live with it.' That did not resonate with my psyche. Up to then I had been a fit and active 57-year-old with a background of fitness and dance, and I wanted to return to this. On finding a cardiologist who specialised in TTS, he organised further diagnostics which showed that even six months post-attack my heart had still not recovered and required two cardiac ablations.

Knowledge is improving but sadly today there still remains a misconception of takotsubo being a benign heart condition – a one-off event from which the patient will recover fully within days or weeks. Sometimes this is the case, but often women have ongoing problems and remain symptomatic. Frustratingly due to the condition being misunderstood, it is frequently mismanaged, leading to a poor outcome for the patient. I was lucky in that I found cardiologists who listened and understood.

Everyone's story arc is different, and for me, I made a promise to myself that one day I would find a way to help others, to stop them from falling through the TTS net, as I had almost done. I hope this has been achieved in a number of ways, not only by myself but with some wonderful people I have met along the way. Initially, I set up a TTS support group into which another group merged and, to date, we have almost 4000 members: https://www.facebook.com/groups/TakotsuboSupport.

This led to the development of a dedicated website (www.takotsubo.net) covering not only general information on TTS but the clinical aspect too, specifically for the medical community; my cofounder happened to be a clinician specialising in TTS. Along with two others, I co-authored a paper: 'Takotsubo syndrome: voices to be heard', which was published in the *European*

*Journal of Cardiovascular Nursing*. My latest venture, along with two fellow patients, is the setting up of a new heart charity, Women's Heartbeat, which specifically aims to improve women's heart health and cardiac outcomes, by raising awareness of women's heart problems via early diagnosis; as well as providing information, education and guidance for both patients and medical professionals, and promoting clinical research into heart disease in women. (www.womensheartbeat.com).

Juliet's story is an honest and at times painful account of her TTS cardiac journey. She wears her heart on her sleeve (excuse the pun) and shares openly the background of her earlier life, through to her heart failure. She describes the pathway of the build-up of trauma over the years, culminating in the more recent two very painful incidents which were perhaps the straws that broke the camel's back. There will be readers who can resonate with cumulative stress (who lives a totally stress-free life?), see similarities and appreciate Juliet's honesty. Juliet illustrates how in some cases, buried and/or ongoing or sudden stress can change one's life course in an instant and affect one's heart to the point when it becomes stunned, is unable to beat correctly and these events result in the heart failing.

Dr Gupta and Professor Dawson's interviews in the book give their expertise and insight into this fascinating, often undertreated condition, and the stories other patients share reflect different causations, journeys and how some have been lucky enough to find consultants who understand the condition whilst others have been cut adrift.

It is becoming more common knowledge that women continue to be second-class citizens when it comes to heart health per se, let alone with a condition that predominantly occurs in women. Women's healthcare needs to now expand beyond the 'bikini medicine' model – i.e. the areas a bikini covers, the breasts and the reproductive area. There is a difference between men's and women's hearts. There is still a bias towards diagnosis, treatment and research in favour of men. There is most definitely a communication issue with regards to TTS.

Hopefully, by patients being outspoken, educating themselves and disseminating information, it will help them to identify what needs to be unlearnt – that TTS is not a trivial condition – and to re-learn what needs learning: that it can be a life-threatening condition and needs to be taken seriously. Books such as Juliet's can help to socialise this information; we need to utilise as many sources for change as possible so that people understand this condition, leading to better education and outcomes.

With health and happiness,

Caron Curragh

PS – A week after writing the above Foreword, the behaviour of the same neighbour caused me to have another TTS episode, demonstrating that recurrence can unfortunately happen.

# Acknowledgements

Thank you to my sister, Karen, who has shared most of this twisting, turning rollercoaster with me, and is one of the few who understand the turbulent and mixed-up emotions that come from complicated mothers and complicated grief.

Thank you to my friend Mia, who not only continues to support me unequivocally throughout my life's trials and tribulations, but who gave me the idea to write about this one.

Thank you to my publisher, Georgina Bentliff of Hammersmith Books, who believed in this book from the moment I emailed her from my hospital bed, and for giving me free rein in its conception and creation.

I am very grateful to the Facebook group I found; as well as offering support, almost all of the information I gathered about TTS in the early days of my diagnosis came from the people in that group.

Thank you to the inspirational Caron Curragh, who wrote the Foreword for this book and whose commitment to giving a voice to women with heart disease is inspiring and very welcome to those of us who have struggled to find the information and support we need.

Thank you to Professor Dana Dawson, whose ongoing dedication to takotsubo is impressive and very much appreciated, and for her extreme generosity with her expertise and insight; as well as to Dr Gupta, for his continued support of women's heart health, and for his kindness in sharing his valuable time and knowledge.

Thank you to all the ladies (and one man!) who shared their stories for inclusion in the book. Their contribution has been invaluable.

To the friends and family who helped me through this, the toughest of times – whether it was providing an ear, a bed for the night, a text or a hug – you know who you are and I am so eternally grateful for your support.

And to Lee, Kerri, Liam, Tom and Dacre. You are my inspiration for all that I do; thank you for your love and care; it has made my heart whole again.

# A note from the author

In 2018 I wrote a book about my 'journey' with gallstones, after being struck down with those odious little nuggets of pain, and for some reason being compelled to tell the world about them. Well, here I go again: writing a book about yet another condition that has suddenly surfaced in my life. I guess that's the way it works with health – one day you are going about your business, taking your wellbeing for granted, blissfully unaware of your body's sneaky little plans; the next minute you are confined to a hospital bed surrounded by people in blue coats with needles in their hands.

This new condition I have has lots of names – don't ask me why. It's like they (by *they* I mean the people whose job it is to give these things names) can't agree. Well, actually, that is a fact: *they* can't agree. After being told in the hospital that I had 'broken-heart syndrome', and then posting about my experience on an online forum, I was quickly reminded that the term was not popular, and was in fact frowned upon. I was told: 'Some of us feel that calling it "broken heart syndrome" detracts from the serious nature of the illness. We prefer to call it "apical ballooning syndrome", or "takotsubo cardiomyopathy".' (A *takotsubo* is an octopus-trap in Japanese. Yes I know that doesn't really explain anything… be patient).

I understand why some people don't like the term *broken heart syndrome*. It would appear to trivialise the condition, making it seem almost whimsical. (After diagnosis, one friend asked me if

I had made up the illness. Fair enough; it admittedly does sound … well, made up).

Also, it is misleading. Takotsubo – or TS or TTS for short (even the acronyms are confused) – is not necessarily caused by an emotional event, which is what *broken heart syndrome* might suggest. As you will learn from some of the stories in Chapter 14 of this book, where others share their experiences, there are a multitude of reasons why people are stricken with it, including near-drownings, conflict, illness, car accidents, major disasters and loss. Confusingly, it can also be triggered by positive events, such as a lottery win or promotion. And sometimes (in fact, in almost a third of cases) there appears to be no trigger at all.[1]

The problem for me is, when three doctors come to me and tell me that I have 'broken heart syndrome', it is hard to dismiss the term. And in *my* case, *broken heart syndrome* describes exactly what I have.

As such, I use the term liberally throughout this book, but with the caveat that I acknowledge it is a misnomer.

You should know, and actually you may already have concluded, that I am not a doctor. Not only am I not a doctor, but I am no kind of health practitioner. I am not an expert in this, or anything, really.

I include a few facts and figures, but as this condition is a relatively new (or rather, newly acknowledged) and rare (as far as we know) one, what we do know about it is evolving, if slowly, and any research I allude to here is some of what is known *to date*. As a non-medical person, I try to make sense of it and relate it to you here in simple terms – this is a reflection of my limited brain capacity, not yours.

I personally knew nothing of takotsubo before I was confronted with it, and I'm not alone in this. Few people know about it – even some doctors – and as such there seems to be some catching up to do, not just by the general public but by some of those in the medical field too.

## A note from the author

Before we go on, I feel I should explain the octopus reference: in the early 90s, a Japanese doctor, Dr Hikaru Sato, was the first to name the condition when he noticed that the heart, when damaged by TTS, took on the shape of and resemblance to an octopus pot. In Japan, *takotsubo* is the name for an octopus trap, hence the name 'takotsubo cardiomyopathy'.

My intention for this book is to contain suggestions rather than advice; anecdotes rather than case studies; and overall positivity rather than gloom and fear. Speaking of which, please do not take me too seriously. My story is not an easy one to tell – among other things, I will be recounting my mother's suicide – and the only way for me to tell it is with a tinge of humour. I believe in the power of laughter. And so, I hope my grim and (literally) heart-breaking story makes you smile a little.

(Having said that, I fully recognise that takotsubo is no laughing matter. It is, in fact, very serious, and I do address that side of it within these pages. Please understand though that this is my story, and as such is not in any way meant to belittle anyone else's experience.)

As a writer, I would rather not be making a career based on tragedy and illness, but we have to make the best of what we're given. On that note, please watch out for my next medical event; I fully expect to make this a trilogy. I am joking.

*Juliet*

# PART I

## Home is where the (broken) heart is

# Introduction

My heart breaks one Thursday in October 2023. I am not being dramatic when I tell you this. I *literally* have a broken heart.

I don't much like *having* a broken heart as much as I like saying it; having it is inconvenient and irritating. It is also life-changing and not in a good way. But let's face it – *saying* that I have an actual broken heart makes me interesting... like I will always have a more fascinating ailment than most of the people I meet; like I will have guaranteed dinner party conversation. Now, that sounds like a dinner party you can only wish to get an invite to.

I don't (or rather, I didn't) consider myself generally anxious or stressed. My emotions are usually kept firmly in check, where, as an English person, I was taught to keep them. (This could be a clue to my condition, but more of that later. Bet you cannot wait.)

And I wouldn't say I have a particularly stressful life. I live on the beautiful west coast of Canada, with my laid-back husband and a cat. Cats are essential for stress management, as are laid-back partners. I am surrounded by good people whom I love. I manage to spend a lot of time in Brighton, England – my home town, one of my most favourite places on earth, where I have a whole network of more people whom I love. I practise yoga daily. I eat fairly healthily (though I do love chocolate, and wine). Basically, I don't have it too tough.

## What becomes of the broken-hearted

This Thursday in October of 2023 though – and come to think of it, the whole of 2023 to this point – has been a bit stressful. Actually, that may be a little bit of an understatement.

After diagnosis, the doctor says to me that I have a 'textbook case of *broken heart syndrome*', and what I think that means is that if someone was to write a guide or textbook on how to get the condition (please don't buy that book), they would describe exactly what this particular Thursday in October consists of.

But before we get to that, I have to take you back to the days when my heart was whole and intact; the days of my unbroken heart.

# Chapter One

# Before the heartbreak

*August 2022*
*Southern England*

We are at a music festival. Only England can do music festivals like this: quirky, vibrant, diverse, full of colour and exuberance.* Living in Canada for the last 20 years has robbed us of the music festival scene, and so we soak it up, Husband Lee and I. It is one of the things we miss about living away from our homeland. I say *we* but I mean *I*; Lee doesn't live his life the way I do, hankering after places or things. He doesn't have takotsubo syndrome either. Just saying.

We arrive at the festival en masse, a group of friends that includes our grown-up daughter and her soon-to-be-husband, bags stuffed with hidden gin and tonics. We might be middle-aged but we still know how to party on the cheap.

As we dance and drink and laugh and sing, I feel lucky to have a group of friends in two countries. I have managed over the past

---

*Sweeping statement/unnecessary patriotism alert! I love to claim that England does things better than anywhere else, but please know that I am not as arrogant as I may seem (although Husband Lee may disagree. Rude.)

20 years to keep my best friends in England, while cultivating a whole new friendship group in Canada. It is one of the things I am most proud of as an expat.

Being an expat has not been easy for me. For those 20 years I have kept one foot planted firmly in both countries, and that has ensured a level of constant homesickness, financial ruin and exhaustion that only an expat, or perhaps a convict, will understand. Or maybe I have just been spectacularly bad at it: never fully committing to living in Canada; hanging on to my English roots; never really letting go, like a mother fiercely clinging to her child well into adulthood. (Oh wait, I do that too. I am the mother who still needs to know where her 35 and 26 year-old 'children' are at all times.)

But there is also a level of excitement about it, in an emotionally and financially draining way. The frequent flying across oceans; the relentless emotional goodbyes at airports; the constant change. It's a jet-set lifestyle, in this case without the glamour or exotic destinations. Mine is the kind of jet-set lifestyle where I am permanently broke, exhausted and in a state of unrest. Yet I thrive on the thrill of it all. I am a dual citizen in every sense.

But in this, the summer of 2022, as I take yet another foray into my 'other' life in England, I have no way of knowing that it will be the weekend when my two worlds will collide, and set about the process of breaking my heart.

Lee and I are here for a friend's wedding. I am also here to indulge the things I miss: my friends and family, obviously; but also British pubs, British shops, British music. You get the picture. The festival is in Portsmouth on the south coast. Scottish singer/songwriter Paolo Nutini headlines the Saturday night and while I 'sing' along to his beautifully soulful tunes, I think about my music-loving friend Susan, who is 5000 miles away in Canada; she would *really* like to be here right now. We have plans for her to come to England in May 2023 for Daughter Kerri's wedding and she regularly asks me to send her snippets of British life. I'll send her a video of me singing along to Paolo tomorrow, I think to myself. She'll love it.

We are staying in a house close to the festival, and when we finally get back there, after meandering through the streets, still buzzing with festival-goers and late-night revellers, it is 1:00 am. 5:00 pm in Canada. Lee is sitting up in bed, and as I get ready to join him, I notice that his face is white, stricken. He is staring with wide, glassy eyes at his phone.

And then he says, 'Oh, no'. Two small words that strike fear into my heart. I stare at him, holding my breath. He looks up at me and says quietly, 'It's Susan'.

My reply is 'Susan who?' – playing for time while my mind starts racing through all the Susans we know. Because I know in this moment that I have lost a Susan.

'Susan A-,' he says. I gasp, without knowing the rest of this story, not wanting to know it. This Susan is one of the best people I know; a one-off; a beautiful, funny, brave woman; a loyal friend, not just to me but to many people. This Susan – mother of three young adults – recently sold her house so she could buy a van and travel around Canada indulging her adventurous spirit. This Susan is excited about coming to England next year, to Daughter Kerri's wedding.

Lee says, 'She drowned,' the words so harsh, so final. So improbable. My first reaction, predictably, is disbelief. This is not possible. Susan is fit, healthy, a strong swimmer, a strong woman;

the least likely woman to have drowned today. And then, as it slowly dawns on me, the realisation that this news is not a lie, or a bad joke, or simply *wrong*, fills me with an indescribable and all-consuming wave of shock. I scream, I collapse. For hours, my body won't stop shaking. It is strange how your body takes over so absolutely in sudden trauma.

There are points in our lives that define us; the befores and afters. The forks, the bends, the lines that are drawn. This is one of those times for me. And as my brain tries to process the reality that Susan has gone, I somehow know that my world will shift on its axis tonight, and it will never again be the same. I have never lost a friend before. I keep repeating this fact out loud, as if it is relevant, or has any meaning. It doesn't, but the fact of it is somehow jolting; another layer of shock that I cannot process.

We go back to Brighton, and the next few days are a blur. I carry on with my life in a country that never knew her, and somehow this mutes the reality, but also makes my grief a lonely place to be. At night I lie awake with thoughts of her in my head – memories, of course; but also imagining and trying to understand her unexplained death; feeling deep sorrow for her daughter and two sons; wracked with a sense of absolute and total loss. I wonder in these long nights how anyone survives grief; it consumes our bodies and minds so completely. It feels to me like I have been swallowed by it; like I have fallen suddenly down a deep, dark hole from which there is no escape.

After three days, one of my best friends, Mia, invites Lee and me to her house, a house that has for the past 20 years felt like a second home to me. It was the house where we spent our last night before we emigrated; it was the place my dad dived into the swimming pool to rescue one of the family rottweilers; it was the site of countless memorable parties and dinner parties; it was a refuge to me after my dad died, after my dog died, after I had my gallstones operation. I welcome its familiarity.

As we sit down to dinner my phone rings. I see my mum's name and sigh heavily. I have changed the contact details on my phone from 'Mum' to her name; a small, private protest. My mum is a complicated woman.

When I had told her about Susan the day before, her reaction was to look uninterested and say nothing. Not one single thing. To be honest I hadn't expected much – I had long ago given up expecting sympathy or interest from my mother – probably since the day my dad died and her words of 'consolation' to me were: 'Well, he was a shit father anyway', but the coldness in her eyes after being told about one of my best friends dying was jarring, even for jaded little old me.

I consider not answering the phone, but I have this masochistic need to subject myself to the anger my mother stirs in me. It is like an addiction. The first sound I hear from her is a sob. I am used to this. I wait for her to speak, and when she does, her voice is flat. 'Are you at Mia's?'

*You know I am.* Deep breath.

'Yes, we are just having dinner," I say. She is not happy to hear this, and I know it. I can sense the envy coursing through the phone line, stealing my energy. If she is not included, she doesn't want to know about it. She certainly doesn't want me to enjoy it.

After a long silence, she says this: 'If I had the right pill, right now, I would kill myself.'

I gasp, though not with sadness or shock. I am infuriated –

incensed – at her cruel disregard for my grief. But I am so exhausted from that grief that I cannot find the energy to release my anger. Instead, I swallow the torrent of words that start to form in my throat, and I take another deep breath – this one as deep as a breath can be – and then calmly say all the 'right' things. What are the right things to say to a pseudo-suicidal mother? Somehow I find them:

'Tomorrow is another day';
'Try to get some sleep';
'I'll come over to take you out tomorrow'.

I put down the phone and return to my dinner, tucking the rage away in a deep recess where the anger of 50 years resides.

The three people I am with (Husband Lee, Mia, and her husband) have heard this all before; when I relay my mother's words there is no shock from them, just a resigned acceptance that she will not allow me to have an evening with my friends without placing herself at the centre of it. And she certainly will not let me grieve for Susan; she wants me to grieve for her instead.

She doesn't have a pill, and she doesn't kill herself. I had known this would be the case of course. But the next day, the guilt creeps in. It is an insipid, evil emotion, this guilt I carry. It fills my head with its accusations: I am a bad daughter. I don't care/help/talk to her enough. I abandoned her to move to Canada. I should have delved more into her suicidal ideation. I should have comforted her. I should have mothered her.

My mother has alienated many people in her life. She writes people off if they have wronged her in some way; usually the ways they have wronged her are imagined, or exaggerated. But in my moments of guilt, or forgiveness, or love, I defend her; there are so many reasons why she is the way she is: she is old;

she has a worsening eye condition – macular degeneration – which has made her almost blind; she is a recovering alcoholic; she is mentally ill; she has had countless rounds of electric shock treatment; she has been sectioned twice; she has been institutionalised long-term, more than twice.

But I, too, am damaged. I am damaged from the years of my mother's alcoholism and illness; from the lifetime of regret, sadness, fear; from my parents' toxic relationship. I was 9 when they divorced; 13 when Mum tried to take her own life the first time (during my lifetime); 15 when she came out of the mental hospital where she had become a frail shell of a woman. I bury those memories deep, too deep for my own good.

# Chapter Two

# Digging deep: tales from a troubled childhood

1975
Brighton, England

I have very few memories of my life before this night. I don't know if I just have a really bad memory, or if my life up until I was 9 was just really boring; not worth remembering. I suppose it is more likely that the trauma of it all erased almost all that had gone before, like I'd had a bump on the head, and just like that, those nine years evaporated.

And so my childhood begins here, on this night, the night before my family dissolved; the night when my dad lay crying between my sister Karen and me in my parents' bed. The sight – and sound – of his sobbing was shocking. At some point he stopped crying and fell asleep, but I lay there for hours, awake and frozen, in a state of confusion and guilt, until the morning shone its harsh and ugly light back into my fractured world.

The evening before, Mum and Dad had sat Karen and me down, told us they were separating, and asked, 'Which one of us do you want to live with?'

'Great question!' I responded brightly. 'Thanks for asking! I mean, obviously we would prefer to live in a stable, two-parent household, but should that not be a possibility at this time, then I think, speaking on a practical level, and on behalf of both Karen and myself, I feel that we should probably opt to live with the parent who has the emotional and financial capacity to bring up two pre-pubescent girls!'

I didn't say that; I was 9. What I did was stare at them both in horrified silence, my voice twisted in my throat, whilst Karen sobbed quietly beside me. At one point I felt hot wet tears sliding down my face, but I wiped them away quickly. I knew that this was a big day for us as a family – a turning point of some kind – and I knew I was expected to be grown up about it, because that's what they kept telling us we should be, but I didn't feel grown up; I felt small, and inconsequential, and scared.

At some point in the proceedings it was agreed between the parties that Karen and I would stay with our mother, though I don't remember being one of those parties. I don't remember agreeing to anything. In retrospect, I suppose my silence was my complicity. Hence the twisting vines of guilt that crept like a slithering snake into my young, undeveloped brain that night, and have never left.

The next day, my red-eyed father left the house carrying three black bin bags, like he was taking out the rubbish, and we didn't see him again for two years.

Because I have a tendency towards the dramatic, I would later claim to anyone who would listen that if I had a chance to go back to that night, and I was asked that question again ('Who do you want to live with, Juliet?'), I would probably not have been silent. I would have probably screamed from the rooftops, as loudly as my little voice could carry me: *'Please.... anything, anyone, but her!'*

Her. My mother. Margaret. When I was born, she said, 'Oh, I wanted a boy'. Which would be funny, if she hadn't repeated this to me regularly throughout my life. The last time she said this to me was shortly before she died. There was nothing in her childhood to suggest the chaos in her mind that was to come later.\* She had a well-balanced, lower-middle-class upbringing with loving parents and two younger brothers.

She met and married my dad when she was in her mid-twenties, when she was a dark-haired voluptuous siren of a woman. My dad was a handsome ex-racing cyclist with an entrepreneurial, and (according to my mum) philandering, spirit. My dad had gone off to the RAF in Hong Kong as a 'normal young man' according to his mum, but after a near-fatal bout of polio, had returned as a wildly ambitious, money-hungry and egotistical womaniser. My mum was physically strong, strikingly beautiful, yet fragile and vulnerable. Theirs was a passionate but doomed union; a raging tornado colliding with a house built from sugar and sadness. That they stayed together for 13 years was remarkable, but those years were cruel to all of us. I don't think Mum ever recovered.

After Dad left, I stopped washing myself. I only remember this because one day at school I was repulsed by an unknown odour so bad that it made me gag, and some days later a boy I had been

---

\*I have just discovered, on reading my mum's official medical history, that she took her first recorded overdose at 16. I have a faint recollection of her telling me this, but I would have dismissed it at the time as her first foray into attention-seeking dramatics. I wish, with a deep sadness and regret, that I could ask her more about it now.\*\*
\*\*Confused about my feelings for my mum? Welcome to my world.

flirting with, Sean, asked me when was the last time I had had a wash. I was mortified, crushed. But still I didn't wash.*

I had been sporty and popular at school, but the not-washing thing changed all that. Kids are quick to judge, and it turns out they don't much like hanging out with smelly girls, however sporty and popular they are.

We lived in a skinny three-storey house in Brighton that had been bombed in the Second World War and rebuilt in the 60s. It had an air of regret about it, like it was bitter about its history.

I remember orange cabinets in the kitchen, orange curtains in the living room, and I am sure I remember orange carpet. Why so much orange? I hated that house and its orangeness. We lived there for years – around 10 I think – but it never felt like home to me. There was a strange presence there; I always felt like I was being watched or followed. My mum swore that there was a resident poltergeist (which was mine and my sister's fault obviously – seeing as poltergeists were attracted by adolescent girls, according to her).

When I think back to this time, after Dad left, I remember a deep, empty sense of loneliness. I have nothing to compare our new fatherless life to, because I have no memories of the old one, the one where he was in it. My sister says she has no memories at all from any of this time, before or after. Her whole childhood.

Mum's job in a local pub took her away at dinner time and bed time, and the mornings of recovery took her away at breakfast time.

---

*I would like to reassure you (and anyone who knows me) that I did, some time later, return to a personal hygiene routine and no longer have B.O. Most of the time.

## Digging deep

One day after school, we got home to an empty house, which was not unusual, but this time we were both hungry. We searched the cupboards until we found a bag of suspiciously green potatoes which seemed to be growing thin brown spikes. Undeterred by their un-potato like appearance, Karen pulled them from the cupboard and said, 'I can make chips! I've seen Mum do it.' She set about peeling and cutting potatoes, and pouring an alarming amount of fat into a pot, while I watched from afar. I didn't trust the potatoes, nor the bubbling fat that started to spit at her angrily. Suddenly and without warning, a fire erupted from the pan, and Karen was splattered with the boiling fat; she screamed in panic and pain, and I ran away.

I am not great in a medical emergency. I am squeamish and also generally clueless about first aid, something I've never bothered to rectify, because – well, I'm squeamish. My instinct is to run from danger, hence the running away part. I didn't just run off into the distance though; I at least had the presence of mind to run to the pub where Mum worked, which was at the end of our street. She wasn't there. In retrospect, weird. She was meant to be not at home because she was working. Seeing my panic, Mum's boss phoned an ambulance and the fire brigade; things I had not thought to do; you know, because I was a child.

Mum's boss suggested we go back to the house, and she followed me as I ran back, imagining the terrible scene that would greet me when I arrived. Flames were not leaping from the roof, though. A fire engine and ambulance were already outside, and I remember an overwhelming sense of relief, mainly that I would not be the one who had to deal with the situation any longer. Karen was sitting on the front garden wall, her face thankfully obscured by two ambulance men; I wasn't ready to see what I imagined would be her melted face and grotesquely blistered fingers.

One of the ambulance men turned to me and said they needed to take Karen to hospital, and where was our mother? Mum's boss, a glamorous, red-lipped woman with a pile of black hair balancing on her head, led the man away and started whispering at him while he looked at her, then back at us, without speaking.

I sat in the ambulance with Karen, who was by now whimpering slightly, and as they put the siren on, I was grateful that I couldn't hear her any more.

We had been sitting in a hospital room for hours when Mum finally turned up, followed by a man we didn't know, both of them engulfed in a nose-stinging, fiery aroma that we knew well. As Mum demanded answers from the doctor who was unlucky enough to be bandaging Karen's hands, I put my arm around my sister and looked at my feet, unable to look at Karen's face, or anyone else's.

Karen survived the chip pan fire with a few scars to her hands, face and chest, which over time healed, but she said she would never try to cook chips again, and repeated this to two serious-faced women who arrived at our door a few days later, asking her questions that she mostly refused to answer. The older woman, dressed in a bottle-green high-necked blouse (I remember this because I have hated bottle-green and high-necked blouses ever since), turned to me with her narrow, squinting eyes and said, 'Does your mother leave you alone a lot?'

My mother was sitting next to me, glowering. I knew what I had to say ('No, never!') but I felt a rising taste of something bitter in my mouth as I said the words. These early years of my childhood were setting me up for a lifetime habit of pushing the pain down.

Our dad appeared back into our lives one day, unannounced, to pick us up from school. I didn't recognise him, and when he told us to get into his car (a brown Ford Granada) I said this: 'Mum told us not to get into cars with strangers'. I don't know if I said it to hurt him, or if I really meant it. I don't think I could have really meant it, because we did get in the car, and just like that, we had a dad again.

After that, we had a sort of arrangement where we would see him every other weekend, and sometimes he took us away on foreign holidays. I say 'sort of' because it seemed to be quite flexible.

I remember one Sunday, Karen and I sat forlornly at our grandma's window, watching cars drive past and waiting for Dad to pick us up, for what seemed like hours. It probably wasn't hours, but there were some days when he never came at all, so each minute we waited was a minute of lengthening despondency. On this day, we squealed with delight when we spotted the Ford Granada pull up. That car was so exotic to me, despite its colour.

To my mother's absolute disgust, I hero-worshipped Dad, whether he was late, early or simply never arrived, and despite his previous two-year absence. Mum once found a note I had written, which I had hidden behind a mirror in the spare bedroom. 'To whom it may concern' (no-one): 'I wish I could live with my dad. I love him so much.' I don't think I need a therapist to tell me I was hoping Mum would find this note. I mean, a mirror? I don't even have time to unpack the meaning behind that.

She confronted me with the note, red-faced and accusing. 'How do you think this makes me feel?' she spat. I was 11, the words I might have spoken unknown to me then.

As a mother now, I look back on this and see the hurt it would have caused. I was being deliberately spiteful. I am not claiming to be blameless in the sad story of my mother's life.

On this Sunday, Dad took Karen and me walking across the South Downs, a range of rolling hills and lush green countryside running through Sussex. Trampling through long grass and with a hot summer sun high above us, I stumbled over something, and when I looked down, it was a smooth, flat length of wood (the size of a small dog) attached to a long piece of thick string. I picked up the end of the string and started pulling it behind me.

My dad named the piece of wood Fifi, and through a high-pitched sing-song voice, he gave it a personality. He spent the rest of that walk entertaining us with Fifi's commentary as I dragged her along behind me, bouncing through the grass. Fifi was English-posh, for some reason.

I know this sounds a bit weird/needy, but I loved Fifi. She felt real to me; alive. I was so excited to take her home and show Mum, who said it was just a bit of old rubbish someone had tossed away.

For the next two visits with Dad, I took Fifi with me, and Dad dutifully resumed his act as her voice and character. We thought it was hilarious when we took her to see a film (*Abba, the movie*) and Dad had her singing *Dancing Queen* at our regular café (Wimpy) afterwards.

A few days after this excursion, I came home from school to find Fifi missing from her usual spot on my bed. I frantically searched my room, upturning bedding and clothes, looking under furniture, becoming increasingly panicked, until the slow realisation of Fifi's fate brought grief-stricken tears to my eyes.

Fifi had been thrown away after all.

Sobbing and looking for – what? Comfort? An admission? – I found Mum in the room next to mine, sitting at her dressing table, a cruel smirk playing on smoke-cloaked lips, dark-rimmed eyes fixed on her reflection, her silence and refusal to make eye contact a dare to my confused anger.

Full disclosure: this memory of my mother is hazy, as hazy as the smoke-filled rooms of my childhood. This memory is likely imagined; born from the feelings I had at the time, rather than the reality. It is more likely that my mum wasn't even there that day.

Look, I know I sound slightly unhinged. I know we are talking about a bit of wood on a string here. But the fact that I am still talking about it, almost 50 years later, and it can still bring a tear to my eye, is a clue to the impact this had on me. The casual discarding of Fifi felt so significant that it is one of the only memories that has survived from those years.

And so it was that my mother became the villain of my childhood.

# Chapter Three

# A silent witness to mental illness

I was 13 when Mum tried to kill herself. I let myself into the house on a Friday evening after school with the familiar feeling I had when I walked through that front door: a sense of dread and sadness. I knew Karen wasn't home; she had stayed at school for some reason. I was planning to spend the evening reading. Books were my saviour back then.

The front door opened to a small hallway on the lower floor, where there was a sparsely furnished family room, the orange-hued kitchen with a door leading to a small grassed garden, and a narrow, white-tiled bathroom to the side. Mum's bag was lying on the floor of the family room, some of its contents spilling out onto the cold wooden floor. Something didn't feel right. 'Mum?' I called out. No answer.

The bathroom door was locked, but there was silence behind it. 'Hello?' Nothing. 'Mum?' I felt a panic start to rise in my gut. Images and memories started to race through my mind. What had happened this morning before I left for school? Nothing; I hadn't seen her – she'd still been in bed. What happened last night? I hadn't seen her then either; she had been out.

Weirdly (because it didn't really seem like the appropriate time) at that moment I started to wonder why I hardly ever saw her. It was such an accepted part of my life, my mother's absence from it, that I rarely questioned it.

I started to push on the door. It gave way quickly (I was not captain of the girl's hockey and netball teams for nothing). As the door crashed open, a repugnant stench hit my nostrils – it was a mixture of sick and alcohol – and I saw a scene that made no sense: the bathroom was empty, but there was a trail of dried-up vomit stuck to the side of the bath, and an empty pill bottle standing upright in its midst. I was confused until it slowly dawned on me that my mother had taken an overdose. And then, I had this thought: 'My mum is dead'. I remember nothing of the rest of that day.

I later learned what had happened. Grandma – Mum's mum – had a 'bad feeling' when Mum didn't answer the phone that morning. She jumped on a bus, used her key to enter the house, and found her daughter in the bath fully clothed, her head resting on the side of the bath, eyes closed, a trail of thick white liquid oozing from her mouth.

By the time the ambulance arrived, Grandma had found Mum's pulse, and sat sitting holding her hand, not knowing if she would live or die. Before jumping in the ambulance with Mum, Grandma had locked the bathroom door from the outside, trying to protect Karen and me from what we would find when we returned home.

In the days afterwards, I felt a sense of terror that my mum would die, and confusion because I could not comprehend how a mother could choose to leave her children, or knowing that one of her teenage daughters would find the aftermath of that choice. But mostly I felt anger, because I suspected that was somehow a part of the impact she was hoping for.

## A silent witness to mental illness

Nobody bothered to explain mental illness to me.

For eight months after that, our mother lived in a psychiatric hospital ward named 'H Block', a nondescript and yet somehow graphically vivid name that chilled our young hearts, and even now, can chill my old one.

Karen and I visited her once a week; it was too hard on us to go more often than that. We would walk past rows of metal-framed beds containing the listless bodies and vacant faces of a hundred lost souls, until we reached our mother, a long-term patient afforded the luxury of a bedside window at the end of the ward.

She would greet us with large, sad, pleading eyes, harshly magnified by unfamiliar and ugly spectacles, set on her bony cheeks, an unsettling silence as she grasped our hands, a look of hopelessness boring into our souls. The stench of cigarette smoke clung to her skin, her clothes, the air around us. She was mostly silent but would sometimes whisper tales of the nurses' conspiracies to steal her soul and her money. She was a beautiful, vibrant woman once, my mother.

We would leave H Block, two despondent, helpless daughters, and the moment we took our first gulp of air from the world outside of that desperate, soulless hospital, we would cry, big bleak tears, on each other's shoulders. For two years, we were lost; two confused teenagers without direction, without a mother, being forced into a harsh and terrifying world of mental illness that we could not comprehend.

We moved in with our dad; his house was cold and sparsely furnished; a true bachelor pad where we found little comfort, emotionally or practically. I suppose I had been wrong to think life would be better living with Dad. He just wasn't equipped to deal with us. It was a strange time; it felt like a chasm in my life, an abyss; like I was subsisting in a nowhere land. I was on auto-pilot, living a teenage life that I have little memory of. But I do remember the constant feeling of fear that followed me for those two years. I feared for my mother's soul; I was convinced she would never recover. I just couldn't imagine how she could.

She did eventually recover, though. But not really, not fully.

We were never told (until later in our lives) about the rounds of electric shock treatment that she endured in that hospital. I asked her as an adult what she could remember about this time, and she said she remembered being lined up like cattle outside a room, about being strapped into a chair and feeling like she had no control over her life. I feel that these memories were not accurate; she probably did not line up outside a room with other people and she was probably not strapped into a chair. But one of the side-effects of ECT is memory loss. And maybe memory loss gets mixed up with images from films and books. I don't know, I'm no mental illness expert. But I wish I had at least *tried* harder to understand it all. I didn't seek the therapy I so clearly needed, but I did run away as soon as I could.

The first time I ran away was to Finland, when I was 16 and found myself living in Helsinki with a much older man who I soon discovered was a paedophile; this is your classic grooming story but it's for another day. I fear I would overload you with sadness/disgust if I tell it now.

Suffice to say, I escaped Finland and the paedophile six months later, after he smashed a rock into my face on a camping trip.

Then, at 23, just after I had Daughter Kerri, I moved to Spain for a year to run a bar. Who doesn't run off to Spain to run a bar when they are 23 and have just had a baby? This was one of the best years of my life, but this could be because it is where I learned to party. That year I lived on Mars bars and vodka.

And finally, aged 35, I ran away to Canada. By this time I had a husband (Lee) and second child (Liam). This move proved to be a bit more permanent than the others. Well, OK, semi-permanent. I don't really do permanent. I don't think it needs a professional therapist to explain this pattern of running away / searching.

And so now, as I write this as a 57-year-old, I am still living in Canada, and I am perpetually confused about that. My heart belongs to England, my soul to Canada. I think. It could be the other way around. When I am in Canada, I yearn for the diversity, personality and culture of England. When I am in England, I yearn for the pristine beauty and the open spaces of Canada. Basically, I am in love with two countries.

I have stayed close to my friends and family since I left – this is not an easy feat when you live 5000 miles apart. I am proud of it; I may have already mentioned that. And despite the lingering guilt I have about leaving, I believe that had I stayed in England, my relationship with my mother would have broken down, possibly irretrievably. It never occurred to me, until now, that maybe, just maybe, I (metaphorically) broke my mum's heart when I left.

In the past 20 or so years, the feelings for my mum have swung like an emotional pendulum, sitting occasionally at the side where hatred lies, hovering briefly in the middle at pity, and swaying all the way to the other side, to love. It is confusing, and exhausting, and it consumes me.

It always has, and I suspect it always will.

# Chapter Four

# Octopus: our safe word

*August 2022*
*Brighton, England*

And so we are back to this day – the day after my mother had made me furious with her cruel disregard for my grief for Susan; for her need to be the centre of attention; and I find myself sitting in her living room and saying: 'Why don't you come and live in Canada for a while?'

I have no idea why I am saying this. When I repeat it later to one of my friends, she looks at me like I have lost my mind and says, 'Have you lost your mind?' Another friend says, 'Do you remember when you told us, just a few months ago, if you ever invite your mum to Canada again, someone should shoot you?'

Yes I do remember this. I remember the way I felt when I said it: exhausted; mentally drained; actually like I could walk away and never look back. I am currently reading a book which talks about cutting off contact with mothers who have narcissistic tendencies and whose presence in their adult child's life can cause more pain than it's worth. People do it all the time – cut contact – to protect their own mental health. But it's never been an option for me. The fantasies I have of cutting contact with my mother are born of frustration and quashed by love and guilt.

So, what's going on here? Why am I asking my mum to come live in Canada, knowing how difficult it will be? Is this my conscience speaking? Am I a masochist? Is it because I know in my heart that one day she will be gone, and I know I must avoid the onslaught of guilt that will undoubtedly come my way? I must not, under any circumstances, give in to this future guilt. I will find a way to retract the invitation.

*December 2022/January 2023*
*White Rock, BC, Canada*

I don't retract the invitation, because I am a cowardly slave to my guilt complex, and five months later, just after Christmas, Mum comes to Canada. Not forever, as I'd suggested, because she says the upheaval is too much (and I agree) but for a month. Which feels like a similar amount of time. Our first argument is on the day she arrives, when she demands my attention and doesn't get it instantly.

Lying in bed later that night, I cry. I hate myself. *She is old, she is almost blind, she is mentally ill*, I think. But I am so tired. She makes me tired. The constant moaning, the constant losing things, the constant irritation, the snapping at me, the demands, the selfishness, the lack of self-awareness. Writing it all now, it doesn't seem so bad. But it is bad. It was bad.

Mum is in good spirits around others. My friends love her. Random strangers love her. She is quirky and eccentric and chatty. But she saves her moodiness, her aggression, her sharp tongue, for me (and my sister). After a few days of her being irritated by me and me by her, I suggest she goes to an AA meeting. I am a big fan of AA and credit it with saving my mother's life, and possibly a few relationships in her life, but she rarely feels the need to actually attend meetings.

This time she agrees, and as I walk her into the meeting, I feel like a mother dropping off her toddler at a new nursery.

Mum walks into the church hall ahead of me, and demands a cup of tea from the first person she sees. The middle-aged woman looks at her with confusion; with a look that says 'do you think you've wandered into a café?' I explain as carefully as I can that my mum has low vision, but I am thinking to myself that I am not sure how this explains her sense of entitlement. The woman points towards a kettle. I make the tea.

Mum grabs another woman who is standing nearby, and starts requesting front row seats 'due to being hard of hearing'. I cringe.

After a few minutes, the woman inexplicably exclaims, 'Oh I love her!' while I am left feeling annoyed and bemused.

When I go back to pick her up, she is standing outside. 'I am just waiting for Jo,' she says. 'She is coming out to have a cigarette with me.' I find I am in the smoker's corner, my least favourite place to be, waiting to meet another of Mum's new friends. She befriends people easily, albeit temporarily, with her exaggerated humour and eccentric chattiness. She is the kind of woman who is impossible to ignore.

Jo comes out. She's young – in her thirties; wiry blonde-streaked hair spilling out from a baseball cap and towering above Mum's 5'4" frame. She offers Mum a cigarette and Mum says, 'Can you light it for me?' Jo looks confused but does it. I want to say, 'Please do not indulge my mother like this. She seems quite able to light the 30 other cigarettes she smokes in a day.' My intolerance is palpable, even to myself.

Jo starts to chat. AA people love to chat AA. I am grateful for it, even if I have heard it all before. Mum says that she is seven years sober and Jo says, 'You have beaten the obsession, well done. Now you need to do the steps.'

Mum says, 'I have never felt the need to do the steps.'

Jo says, 'We all need to do the steps. Without the steps you will always be irritable, restless and discontented.'

When we get to the car, Mum asks me, 'Do you think I am irritable, restless and discontented?'

'Yes,' I say. Easiest question I have ever had to answer.

She is visibly bruised. 'It's my eyes,' she says sadly, and I soften.

'I know how hard it must be to deal with being unable to see properly,' I say. I avoid saying, 'You have had eight years to get used to it,' because that would be cruel. Instead I say this: 'Susan would like to have your problem, though. She would give up her eyesight to be alive. She was 53 with three young adult children, and she is dead. You just have to make the best of it, Mum. Not making the best of it doesn't serve you.' Maybe this is equally cruel.

She turns to me with a flash of rage in her eyes. *'Doesn't serve you?'* She is mocking me. 'What does that mean?'

'It means, Mother, that you can choose what to be upset about!'

## Octopus: our safe word

I feel the familiar rage bubbling, but I don't want it. I don't want this fight. I come up with a genius plan.

'Why don't we have a safe word, Mum? If either of us starts to feel angry or upset, one of us says the word and it will distract us, and remind us not to argue.'

She likes this idea. 'How about the word "octopus"?' she asks. I agree. I feel like progress has been made. I frantically start texting my sister telling her a corner has possibly been turned. Twelve minutes later, standing in my kitchen, for absolutely no reason she says this: 'You are always putting me down.' I am enraged, because this accusation is not true, and is unjustified. I despise injustice, and so I over-react. I scream at her, 'What exactly have I said to make you say that?'

She is shocked by my reaction and so she shouts, 'Octopus!'

'No!' I snap. 'Saying "octopus" will not end this conversation. You cannot accuse me of something I haven't done, and then leave me with it.'

This is one of those things that is a weird and inexplicable coincidence. Why the word 'octopus'? A word that would, 10 months later, have so much significance in my life.

Inevitably, I feel guilty. I should have just kept my mouth shut. Trying to evoke any kind of accountability from her is futile. I don't understand why I don't ever learn. And I don't understand, now, why I didn't try to talk this through; why I didn't try to see my own culpability.

I go to bed. I spend a lot of time in my bed while Mum is here. I am mentally drained. Once again, I feel a fleeting wish that I could go to sleep and not wake up. It is not that I want to die; I just feel so tired, so guilty, so ill equipped to constantly deal with this emotional rollercoaster. It feels so unfair to Susan, this casual disregard for life. I am disgusted with myself for feeling it.

The rest of Mum's trip is an emotional rollercoaster. I try to help her when she needs reassurance; I try to listen without comment when she talks about all the wrongs that have been done to her; I try to give her a sense of hope when she says she sees no future. I feel sorry for her when she tells me she doesn't want to go home, doesn't want to live in her house, doesn't want to be lonely. I again tell her I will look into her coming to live permanently in Canada. And I mean it, even though I know that if she does that, my life will be difficult. No, not difficult; disastrous. I discuss this with a few people who are close to me, and they all agree: I am nuts.

When I drive her to the airport after her three weeks are over, we are silent in the car. In all reality, I am counting down the minutes, but when I hug her goodbye, I say, 'I love you,' and I mean it. I watch her shuffle towards security, small, frail, red-eyed, and the relief I feel is mixed with a profound sense of sadness. As usual, I am confused by my feelings.

As her red hat disappears around the corner, I wave goodbye and unexpected tears trickle down my face. It will be the last time I see her alive.

# Chapter Five

# My mother's suicide

*17th March 2023*
*Canada*

I am doing yoga when the call comes. I don't know why I do yoga. It makes no noticeable difference to anything. After three years of daily practice, I still have thick ankles and no discernible waistline. But I like it, and as I fold my 57-year-old body into a shape it is not meant to be, I resent the ringing telephone.

I stop mid-fold, and stare at the phone, which is on the mat below me. Instinct tells me that what comes next will change my life.

My mother has not been answering her phone for two days. I can't go knock on her door, seeing as I live 5000 miles away. When I awoke this morning, I called her number again, multiple times. With every unanswered ring, I said aloud, 'She's gone,' but as I said those words, I felt nothing.

And so I answer the phone, knowing in my gut what is coming. But then, when it comes; when I hear my sister crying, when I hear the words, 'Juliet, she's gone,' I do not feel nothing. I feel absolute, gut-wrenching, all-consuming, guttural, physical pain.

The pain is so intense that I scream. I think I am going to throw up. I cannot speak. I manage to say, 'I will call you back,' and then I collapse, sobbing, convulsing, on the floor.

And, for most people, this is probably a natural reaction to being told your mother has died. But, as you know, I have spent the past 20 years living in different countries to avoid this woman. I have spent the past two years regularly claiming out loud that I *can't stand* her. Turns out I could stand her. Turns out the pain of her death is overwhelmingly intense. It is a pain I did not expect.

It's not really that shocking for an 86-year-old, chain-smoking, ex-alcoholic to die. But what *is* shocking; what floors me; what rips out my heart and crushes my soul, is that when I do manage to collect myself and call my sister back, her next words are these: 'She killed herself.'

She killed herself six weeks after returning from her trip to Canada. On the day she took her life, she had returned from a visit to the doctors, accompanied by Sister Karen, where the GP listened to her saying how desperate she was, and had then asked her, 'Are you suicidal?' to which Mum replied, 'I want to die, but I am not going to do anything about it'. The GP said she would refer her to the mental health team. Mum, I imagine consumed with hopelessness, went home and took a shit load of pills, took herself to bed, and ended the perpetual mental anguish that defined her life.

The weeks preceding that day had been traumatic. Mum had gone home from Canada and fallen into a deep depression. She told me on the phone that she was struggling to make any decisions in her life. She knew she needed help but she said her head felt muddled. This was not surprising; she had not eaten properly in two weeks. The week before, I ordered some ready meals online and had them delivered. She told Sister Karen to take them away. Karen and I agreed she needed outside help. I tried to get care for her from the council. I called them; I emailed them; I filled out forms online, telling them it was urgent. I never heard back from them.

Karen found a residential care home that had experience with mental health and would take her in temporarily, to care for her and protect her from herself. She took Mum to see the home. It was lovely, more like a hotel.

Afterwards, on the phone, I told Mum that we felt it was best she went into the home short-term until we could sort out more permanent care. And I told her, 'I am still looking into you coming to live here in Canada'. I meant it.

She ranted and rallied and told me she didn't want to go into a home and never had. But Karen and I persisted and eventually she gave in. 'OK, I will go,' she said, but then she said, 'It's so expensive though, it will eat into your inheritance'. I said, 'Mum I don't care about that. We just want you to be safe'. I told her I didn't care if she spent all her money on being looked after, and I meant that too.

'I just can't seem to make any decisions,' she said, and I replied, 'You don't need to. Karen and I will make them for you.'

I regret those words. I thought I was reassuring her, but I wasn't. I was taking away her power. I was also suggesting that we would put her in the home, whether she wanted to go or not.

Mum liked to tell a story, of when she had visited a clairvoyant years before who had told her that her daughters would look after her in her old age, and that when she relayed the conversation to me, I had said, 'You are wrong. We will be putting you in a home as soon as we can.'

And we would laugh and she would make me promise I never would. Hahahahaha, hilarious stuff. Hilarious, heart-wrenching, achingly tragic stuff.

There I was, telling her we were doing exactly what I had promised I wouldn't.

I spent 45 minutes talking to her but she was manic and I was getting really fed up with it. The last thing I said to her was, 'Mum, I need to go'. I imagine her thinking, 'No, it is me who needs to go. And I will.' And she did.

It was the last conversation I ever had with her.

# Chapter Six

# One funeral and a wedding

*April 2023*
*Canada and England*

And so here I am, sitting on another plane, suspended between two countries, once more crossing the ocean in grief. It feels surreal. I can see my bloated red face in the reflection of the window next to me. There are lines at the corners of my eyes that weren't there a week before; I trace them with my finger. It is shocking what emotional trauma can do to your face. I look 10 years older than I did a week ago. I am stocked up with sleeping pills, and anxiously awaiting the arrival of the drinks trolley. I think to myself, *I am going to end up an alcoholic drug addict – and I don't even care.*

I seem to have adopted this attitude with a kind of warped self-satisfaction. I repeat to myself *I don't care* over and over like a mantra. This is a new feeling for me – I am normally quite upbeat. I feel like I will never be upbeat ever again. I feel like I will not care about anything ever again. How does a person recover from their mother's suicide?

The trouble with sitting on a plane between Canada and England is you have nine hours to contemplate, or in my case spiral. The medication and alcohol probably don't help, but my mind is so clouded and my heart is so heavy that I sit here wishing the plane would crash and end my misery. Although that does seem a little selfish considering there are 300 other people on board.

Once again, I start to wonder how a person can ever get past grief. It feels so absolute, so overwhelming, so impossibly dark. I am thankful I have a window seat, where I can turn my head away from every other face on the plane. I cannot bear the *reality* of other people, with their oblivious, ignorant smiles and their facile chatter. Look at them, just going about their day like everything is normal!

Grief is such a dark and desolate place to be. Your head is assaulted with memories, good, bad, sad, happy. Shared memories that are no longer shared. Your pain is absolute, with no hope for respite. No painkiller can reduce this level of pain. No sleeping pill can save you from the inevitable onslaught of sadness that will hit you unexpectedly, day or night. I wish you didn't know this but you probably do.

As we come into land in London, the plane soaring over England's endless fields of green, tears spring to my eyes, as they always do. The familiar and overwhelming sense of being home overtakes my senses; with every fibre of my body, I am connected to this place. But this time, the sense of being home is darkened by an ache in my heart, and it physically hurts. This is the first time in my life that I have come home to a home that no longer includes my mother. As the wheels touch down, my eyes and throat sting. I am so sick of crying. I am sick of the physical weight of it. I am dreading the weeks ahead of me, knowing that more tears will come, as unstoppable as a runaway train.

## One funeral and a wedding

Being in England feels right, though. Like I am home. I go to Mum's house, expecting an onslaught of pain. As I turn the key in the lock, I steel myself for the sadness that will engulf me. But what I feel as I walk through the door is pure anger. It is physically overpowering; it starts in my toes, weirdly, and slowly creeps upwards throughout my whole body. As soon as I feel it rising, I can sense my muscles clenching along with my fists. And then I start to punch things. Not really hard things like walls or doors though; that would be silly. I punch cushions and beds and cuddly toys; things I can't damage and things that can't damage me. I am guessing this punching thing is like a physical release; a way for my body to cope. And I say things like, 'You stupid cow!' out loud. A way for my anguished brain to cope. I would often call my mum a stupid cow to her face; it was a joke, most of the time. It is not a joke now. She would laugh when I insulted her. I will never have that kind of relationship with anyone else in my life.

In 'my' bedroom, the one where I stay on some of my trips to England, but only if I have no other options, I find a framed photo of Husband Lee and me; it is stuffed in a drawer, face down. I find the birthday card I sent her a month earlier, hidden behind a sofa. These discoveries take my breath away. She must have really felt that I failed her at the end.

I force myself to go into her room, abandoned remnants of her life just left scattered there for me to find: reading glasses on the floor beside her bed; half-smoked cigarettes resting on the side of an ashtray, on her bedside table; framed photos on the walls, of her, of us, of Karen, of her grandchildren.

I stare at the nicotine-stained walls, the dust-covered ornaments, the countless butterflies on the walls (how did I never notice before that she collected butterflies?), discarded papers (but no note), and finally I stare at her single bed, the bed she has slept in for the past 15 years. A symbol of loneliness, now a grave. A tiny pink and crystal chandelier hangs above the bed and when I look at it, cobwebs cloak it like a horror film prop. A word springs to my mind: macabre. The scene of my mother's death is macabre.

I stay in England for nine weeks. My first job is to plan my mother's funeral, along with Sister Karen. This is a strangely cathartic process. Writing a eulogy, planning music, food, speeches, karaoke. If anyone is going to have karaoke at their funeral, is it our mum.

I sail through the funeral. In fact, I put this day into my 'Jar of Joy'.*

Mum gets everything she wanted – she had of course pre-planned most of her funeral years ago. We sing, dance, cry, laugh. She would love to be here.

At the funeral, someone comes up to me and says, 'What a lovely mum she was'. 'Thank you' gets stuck in my throat, because all I want to say is, 'How can a mum be lovely if she chooses to leave her children?' I love her, I miss her, I wish she wasn't dead, but I am so full of anger. I cannot forgive her for leaving like this; I cannot get past it. I don't understand why people aren't saying to me, 'What a wicked and selfish thing your mum did'. I suppose people don't say things like that at a funeral.

The reasons for my anger are obvious: my mother took away my chance to say goodbye, my chance to help her; but she also didn't

---

*My Jar of Joy is a small jam jar stuffed with slips of paper describing amazing events that happen to me throughout the year. I have had one for the past five years, though 2022 and 2023 are sparse.

give me a right to reply. And she has ensured that I live with guilt and regret for the rest of my life. I am also angry for what she has done to my kids. Thanks to her, their chances of acting on any suicidal ideation they might have, have statistically increased.[2] I am pretty sure mine have increased too, but I am confident that my occasional wish never to wake up, or to get hit by a bus, are more like fleeting fantasies. I need some better fantasies.

Will I ever stop banging on about anger? It seems like I have lived my whole life with this bubbling rage, and now it will become a part of who I am, maybe the biggest part.

There have been so many phone conversations over the years when she would slam the phone down, after some imagined slight or criticism from me. I was always so enraged, as I was left staring at the silent phone, knowing the words I wanted to say would remain unsaid forever. And now, there will never be another chance to say these words. She has made sure of that.

If I had just played her game, been compliant, been more empathetic, more docile, less argumentative, less combative, she would have felt more validated, more understood, less criticised. I wonder at what cost that would have been. I am not docile; I am reactionary; I am strong-willed and can be defensive. My personality is no more changeable than hers was. Had I been the daughter she might have needed me to be, my head – or maybe my heart – would have probably exploded. But in the aftermath, I regularly awake in the dead of night with this thought in my grief-filled head: *I should have tried harder.*

We could always argue fiercely, and then make up quickly. It was one of the things she said she cherished about our relationship. This time though, she never gave us the chance to make up.

Someone talks about the 'stages of grief', and tells me it is normal to be in the 'anger' stage. I am not a subscriber to the 'stages of grief' thing. I think grief is different for everyone, and I think grieving a suicide is in a league of its own. Not harder than any other grief, just different. I don't think my anger will ever go away. I can't see how it can.

I also recognise that my anger is a comfort blanket. Being angry is better than being sad. I am almost scared for the anger to dissipate.

Funeral over, I need to put my grief, anger and sadness aside as I go full tilt into wedding planning. The funeral is in early April, and Daughter Kerri's wedding is at the end of May.

I don't know if you know this, but planning a wedding is really time-consuming. I throw myself at it like a – well, like a wedding planner. I immerse myself in table plans, colour schemes, name placement tags, and buying stuff. It's almost like I am distracting myself from something.

I mean, I am not claiming I plan the whole wedding – Daughter Kerri (and the actual wedding planner) have done most of it. But the last-minute stuff is relentless. This is a three-day festival wedding so there is a lot to do.

When the wedding comes around, it is incredible; perfect – a fairytale weekend at an English country estate. The speeches mention Susan and Mum and I do not flinch. I do not allow myself to cry. I am resolutely brave.

If my mind starts to wander; if I look at the bedroom that was set aside for Mum – that Kerri does not allow anyone else to occupy – or the single bed in my room that was for Susan, or the places at the tables where the two of them should be, I push down my grief and put a smile on my face, and pick up the nearest glass of champagne.

I am, of course, in denial.

# Chapter Seven

# Back to reality

*June 2023*
*Canada*

I fly back to Canada and predictably fall apart.

I have been in England for nine weeks – nine weeks of my life being on hold; nine weeks of rollercoaster emotions; of extreme sadness and supreme joy. Nine weeks of sleeping in other people's beds, living out of suitcases, cooking in someone else's kitchen, of being away from my cat, my son, my husband (for the most part; son Liam flew to England for the funeral and again for the wedding, Husband Lee came for the wedding). But as I board the plane at Heathrow, I hear my mother in my head saying, 'Leaving so soon?'

In Canada, I struggle to get back to my old life, the one where death and suicide were not lurking in the shadows.

I hole up at home and don't want to leave it. My relationships with people feel tenuous. I have no interest in fluffy conversations. I am craving real, deep, human experience-type connections. And yet I also crave nothing from anyone. I don't laugh as much as I used to. I feel like I have lost myself.

After a few weeks of trying to settle back into my life in Canada, I force myself to go out. I walk through the streets of the small city where we live, White Rock, which nestles on the shores of the Pacific. I am assaulted by memories of when Mum was here just a few months earlier. Cafés where she would demand her tea be served in a tiny china tea cup; restaurants where she would befriend serving staff with her witty charm; a charity shop where the manager asked her to leave because she was being obnoxious; the beach, where she asked a random stranger to take a photo of her climbing onto a sculpture; a pub where she, Susan and I laughed together; the restaurant where she, my friend Shannon and I had our last lunch together; these memories hit me square in the face and leave me breathless.

I prefer, and so desperately cling to, the bad memories – the ones where I can justify my irritation and anger. If a good one comes sneaking in, I quickly banish it. Those ones hurt too much.

Shannon tells me that she frequently sees signs from her dad who passed over a year ago. In fact, a hummingbird visits her most days. My mum loved stuff like that. She will start sending me signs, I decide, and I will get some comfort from that.

Years ago, I read *The Secret* (by Rhonda Byrne) and subsequently went around for weeks declaring that I could attract whatever I wanted into my life. To demonstrate this to Son Liam, I took him and Hallie the dog for a walk to the local park and announced, 'We are going to find a ball. It will be white and blue.' The two of us repeated it like a mantra, until we did, indeed, find a white and blue ball, in a ditch – clear proof that *The Secret* works! It has not worked so well since that day though, despite my many requests for lottery wins and a flat tummy.

But today I decide that I will give it another go. I am ready for a sign from my mother; a symbol of her presence; of her forgiveness; and I will use the long-forgotten powers of *The Secret* to attract it. Walking through the streets of the town, I quietly speak these words: 'Mum, please send me a white butterfly,' and to the universe I say this: 'A white butterfly will land on my arm,' because you have to actually be quite specific about it. I walk and watch, waiting for the butterfly to come. When no butterfly lands on my arm, I realise I might be being *too* specific, so I say aloud: 'A white butterfly will land on a flower near me'. No butterfly appears, so I change it again, to: 'A butterfly (any colour is acceptable) will fly somewhere near me.'

This is about as prime-time butterfly season as you can get. Late summer; an abundance of delicate, wild flowers around; glorious sunshine. Not one single butterfly in sight. It seems less likely that there would be absolutely no butterflies at all during my 45-minute walk, than a white one would land on my arm, and then it hits me: 'Of course! *This* is the message from my mother: "Screw you and you your butterfly demands!"'

I realise that I will probably never get signs from her. She is angry. Typical. *She* is the one who is angry.

I wonder if she is as angry as me; if her anger is as relentless as mine. The rage I carry is more powerful than any other emotion I have. Suicide has robbed me of the 'normal' process of grief, whatever that is. Three months in, I say to Lee: 'I feel so angry; what she did was so selfish.' His response shocks me: 'I disagree. I think what she did was brave.' He continues: 'She was never going to go quietly into the night; she was never going to give in to blindness, or dementia, or any other illness. She was never going to give up her independence.'

These words cause me to reflect and reassess. A bit. I start to let the anger go a little, but what comes after that is much worse. What comes after that is regret. It is regret, I believe, that leads to my heart breaking.

# Chapter Eight

# Be still my broken heart

*12th October 2023*
*Canada*

It is the day of the inquest into Mum's death, and I awake at 5:30 am (an alien concept to me, and quite jarring to my whole being; I am not a morning person; I'm not an any time of day person really – I am just mostly a tired person). The inquest is in England, so I am attending remotely.

I sit up in bed, laptop balancing on my lap, and click the link which has been sent to me by the coroner's office. The court room appears on my screen; it is small and formal, and I can see a TV screen sitting high on a wall in the corner; I am surprised to see my face appear on it. From there I will be observing the proceedings and I think how weird that will be for my sister, my face suspended in the corner high above her, like Kryten's head from *Red Dwarf*. Apologies if you are too young for this reference. (But if you are too young, I recommend you find this TV programme somehow and watch right now. It will be infinitely more entertaining than a book about broken hearts.)

I hastily change the background on my camera so that the court cannot see that I'm in bed in my dressing gown; now they can see my face superimposed on to a static and wholly inappropriate tropical beach. There are palm trees sprouting from my hair, which is flickering slightly; I am a non-talking head looking tired and out of place.

I watch as my sister Karen, her son Freddie and Friend Mia (representing me, supporting my sister) file into the court room. They are smartly dressed and their faces are sombre. This feels surreal, like I am watching a real-life soap opera.

I listen as the coroner does her thing: talks about my mum; reads various reports from doctors, mental health professionals, and my sister – the last person to see her alive.

The inquest is to establish the cause of death, says the coroner. To be honest, none of us really need this; we already know. I had previously asked for Mum's GP to be questioned at the inquest. Neither Karen nor I have been satisfied with her care of our mother, nor her explanations in the aftermath of her death. The coroner asks the GP to take the stand, where she nervously swears an oath. She has brought legal representation, and there he sits beside her, writing furiously in his unseen notebook.

The coroner asks the GP a few questions, and then asks Karen and me if we wish to address her. Karen asks the GP a few more questions, and I hear her voice shaking. The GP's voice is also shaking when she responds.

The coroner addresses me: 'Would you like to ask the GP anything?'

My mind goes blank. After a lot of umms and errs, I compose myself and ask, 'Did the fact that my mum was 85 pounds on the day you saw her ring any alarm bells?'

Also I ask, 'Did you not feel that my mum stating she wanted to die was sufficient reason to refer her for urgent psychiatric assessment?'

I do not remember what the GP replies to either question. I do remember that she is evasive and a little defensive. She would be, I suppose. I try to put myself in her shoes. I don't think it can be easy being a GP; having to know so much about so many things. But I do wonder why some GPs seem to know so little about mental health. And I wonder why this one knows even less than most; a fact that my mum bemoaned regularly. I should have listened. I believe, and this may be unfair, that if my mum had had a different GP, she would still be here.

After the inquest, I Facetime with Karen, Freddie and Mia, and we dissect the experience. I am not distraught, which I'd expected to be; I am numb. We speak calmly. We decide not to continue to aim blame towards the GP. I think this is a form of forgiveness, and with forgiveness comes a lighter burden to carry, I hope.

I say goodbye to the three of them and then I sit in silence with myself, in my empty, noiseless house. I lie in bed afterwards, my laptop still open, staring ahead at nothing in particular, in a kind of blank stupor. It is still only 8:00 am here, but by the time I go down to make my morning coffee I feel like I have lived a whole day. I move around the kitchen like I am swimming through mud; slowly functioning but not really knowing how. I realise that I should have accepted Husband Lee's offer to stay home with me for the day. But I am so strong and independent!

I am the sort of person who likes to get things done. I like to have a purpose; to feel I have achieved something in my day. Most of the rest of this day is spent achieving nothing – wandering around the house, picking things up, putting them down, trying to formulate thoughts from the scrambled mess in my head. At one point I take a break from doing nothing to go outside and walk up the steepest hill in the town. You know, for fun. I am fit and healthy, remember?

When I return, I open my laptop and do some writing. Not for this book, because this book has yet to be born, but for another one, which also talks about my mum's suicide, and my childhood, and other dark and painful memories. My books are so cheery, I bet you cannot wait for the next one. It's tough sometimes to allow myself the space to write what I need to, but today the words come easily; flowing from deep within my soul. I am like a dredger, sucking up all the shit from the seabed and spewing it all out on the page.

And then, as if all these things are not enough, I trot off to my suicide bereavement support group. This is the third week I have attended the group, which is every Thursday for two hours for the next eight weeks. Daughter Kerri affectionately calls it 'Suicide Club'. You have to keep it light when you are dealing with such darkness.

The group consists of two facilitators plus six grieving women, all of whom have lost someone to suicide. I found the group by researching 'local suicide support', and was surprised and saddened to find there are many groups supporting the suicide-bereaved. Surprised because it brings home the reality that there are so many people out there, all going through this hell.

Husband Lee does not understand my need to go to this group; why I have a need to hear the heartbreaking stories of others. The first week was harrowing, with each of us introducing the group to 'their person' and a brief description of how their person died. We bond instantly over our shared trauma. But it is exhausting. I feel each of these women's pain deep in my soul, and when it is my turn, my own pain spills out of me as I talk about the anger I carry and the peace I seek.

And so, to week three. As I drive to the group, I feel detached, like this is someone else's life. Like I am watching it unfold, a spectator on the sidelines. This week we are writing things we wished we had said to our person on scraps of paper, and then burning them in a fire. On mine, I write: 'I wish I had listened to you.' This is a truth that haunts me. My mum was difficult to be around – she was often irritable and self-centred, and her stories were full of self-pity and vitriol towards other people – but still I wish I had listened more. I wish I had asked more. I did try once to record her talking about her life – to help her work through her demons – but it had been a frustrating experience; she had been repetitive and full of blame. I have those recordings on my phone but I don't think I will ever be able to listen to them.

I look at the words I have written; there are only seven of them but they are shocking to me because they are so, so sad; so full of regret. I throw the piece of paper onto the fire and watch as a flame licks at its corners. It starts to curl up into itself; the flame ignites, consumes it quickly, and renders my words to a pile of ash.

Suddenly my heart starts to beat wildly. It's like a tiny person is thumping at the inside of my chest with a hammer. I feel nauseous. Then I start to feel like I can't catch my breath. I sit down heavily, not wanting to make a fuss. These people have enough to deal with; I won't make this about me. The facilitator asks me if I am OK to drive home. 'Yes, of course,' I say with a forced smile.

## What becomes of the broken-hearted

I sit in my car for 10 minutes, breathing heavily and willing the odd feeling in my chest to pass. I manage to drive the 30 minutes home but I don't feel right. When I get back to the house, I have what I can only describe as a desperate need for love; a craving for a giant hug. It feels almost like a primal need. In retrospect, this makes sense. My heart is literally breaking (there I go again with the dramatics), and my body is responding with a cry for help; a request for the one thing it needs – comfort. Husband Lee obliges; wrapping his arms around me tightly and holding me until I start to feel calmer.

He pours me a glass of cab sav, then runs a deep, warm bath (husbands are occasionally quite useful), and there I bask for half an hour, soothed by bubbly water, wine, and love.

Thankfully, I start to feel better, and Lee, Doctor Google and I decide I have had a panic attack, and not even a bad one. I take a sleeping pill and go to bed. I sleep an oblivious seven hours, while my heart changes shape and with every heartbeat starts to restrict the blood flow to the rest of my body.

# Chapter Nine

# Friday the 13th

*Friday 13th October 2023*
*Canada*

Yes, it's Friday the 13th. I am not superstitious, but my mum was. On this, the day I will be diagnosed with a condition named after an octopus pot, I have to wonder, is this whole thing a message from her? Did she arrange it from above? And the reason I have to wonder is because of our safe word. Octopus.

'I'll give you OCTOPUS as a safe word!' I can hear her saying sarcastically. 'How about I give you an octopus-themed health scare instead?' Wahahahah! (aka evil laugh).

I know I am making a leap with this connection. And also I am really not sure if people who are dead are capable of such things. It just seems like such a weird and inexplicable coincidence. And also, just the sort of thing she would do. Come on, even with the little you now know about her, you surely are thinking it too? I admit, I might be over-stretching, but there is something darkly funny as well as strangely comforting about it.

Anyway, I awake on this Friday the 13th and at first I feel fine, if a little tired. I lie in bed for about 10 minutes before getting up to go downstairs to make my morning coffee. I love this routine, the making of the coffee, the taking of the coffee back to bed, the relishing of the extra 20 minutes in bed before facing the day.

But on this day, I don't get to do any of that. As I start to walk down the stairs to the kitchen, with every step I start to notice an increasing feeling of compression in my chest. By the time I reach the kettle, I am panicking, though honestly this is no longer anything like a panic attack. This does not feel good. It feels really bad actually. It feels like nothing I have ever experienced: not pain, as such; more like extreme and overwhelming discomfort mixed with an unnerving sense of dread.

I stagger back upstairs with the intention of getting back into bed, but I can't get there; I fall on the floor on all fours, gasping for breath. I can't seem to get enough air into my lungs. I text Daughter Kerri to ask her to come and help me. She is only downstairs, and I could shout for her, but that seems so dramatic and unnecessary. So I text and wait for a response.

She eventually sees the text and arrives in my bedroom to see me on the floor, white-faced and panicking. You know, as in panic attack. There is simply no other explanation for it. 'I'm having some sort of panic attack,' I tell her.

'I'm calling for an ambulance,' she says.

'No! I am not going to hospital for a panic attack!'

We agree that she can call 811 – the health line. I listen to her explaining the details of what I am going through, again with a sense of detachment from my body.

## Friday the 13th

The operator tells Kerri that we should go to Emergency right away. I reluctantly agree, but I insist we go via the bank, because – well, I have some banking to do.

(This refusal to acknowledge that we are going through a serious problem is something I encounter frequently when speaking to other women who have experienced TTS).

At Emergency, they take the whole thing a little more seriously than me. I am having blood taken soon after arriving, having an ECG 20 minutes after that, and then I am quickly put in a cubicle to await the arrival of a doctor, smug that I have managed to bypass a whole waiting room full of people.

I am starting to feel less breathless, and less panicky, and an hour later when the nurse tells me my ECG is totally normal, I smile a knowing smile at Daughter Kerri and say something like, 'See, I told you'. But the blood results are not in yet, of course. And when they are, everything changes.

The results come back while I am having a chest x-ray. I come out of the x-ray room to find a nurse waiting to take me back to Emergency; she has a quiet sense of urgency about her.

As we approach the cubicle where Kerri waits for me to return, I see another nurse hanging around looking impatient. In one hand she holds a clipboard, and in the other she clutches a huge syringe which she is waving around in the air, like a weapon. (I may have remembered the syringe part wrong.)

As she spies me coming down the corridor, she announces, 'We are moving you to a room!'

'OK, great!' I say enthusiastically. I really like this level of service.

In healthcare terms, it's the difference between flying economy and first class.

I go to pick up my backpack and the nurse swoops past me, skillfully finding room in one of her already-occupied hands to pick up my bag. 'Not you!' she says firmly. This is seriously impressive – even in first class you have to pick up your own luggage.

She ushers me to a private room, still in Emergency. A real bed awaits me and I am instructed to lie on it. Immediately, yet another nurse appears followed by a Young Doctor. They all look serious. I don't have time to process that something serious is actually going on here.

The New Nurse starts preparing my arm for an IV. I do not like needles so I say, 'Why do I need this? What's going on?' There is a tinge of hysteria in my voice.

'It's a precaution,' she says. Weird. Precaution for what?

The Young Doctor looks up from his notes, and I see concern in his eyes.

'Can you run through the events of yesterday for me please,' he says. Once again, I relay the details of my Thursday: the inquest, the walking up the hill, the suicide club, the 'panic attack'. I still think to myself that I am fine.

'As you know, your ECG was normal,' he says, 'But your blood test has shown an elevated level of an enzyme called troponin. What this shows us is that you are experiencing the symptoms of a heart attack.'

I respond with, 'Not possible. I am fit and healthy.' It is true, to an extent. I do eat healthily (I also love chocolate). I don't smoke (but I do love wine). I think I may have already mentioned this. I exercise every day (except when I'm hungover). I have always carried a little extra weight. OK, I am not perfect. But I am also not heart attack material. Or am I?

'That is quite likely,' he says, 'But we suspect what you are experiencing is a condition called takotsubo syndrome, which is also known as broken heart syndrome.'

A solitary tear slides down my face. Yes, just one. For some reason, I apologise on its behalf. The Young Doctor says, 'It is perfectly understandable. You've just been told you're having a heart attack.'

(This is not technically true. Takotsubo is not a heart attack; rather it is a form of heart failure.)

So this is what a broken heart feels like? Not emotional chaos; not lying in a heap on a cold stone floor crying uncontrollably amidst abject sadness and despair. Actual, real physical discomfort. Like a truck is sitting on my ice-cold chest and squeezing the life out of me. Like I can't get my breath; like I have just climbed a mountain in the winter and I am struggling to recover from it.

I am shocked, obviously. Not only is this a condition that I have never heard of, but it is so... not like me. I am not emotionally vulnerable! I am strong! But there is also an element of relief: healing from a broken heart seems like it will be way easier than dealing with *real* heart disease. This is reinforced when the doctor tells me that my condition is 'fully reversible' and I will be recovered within mere weeks, if not days. (In retrospect, I can't help but feel that this was a wild, and potentially erroneous, claim.)

When Husband Lee and Son Liam arrive at the hospital, following a panicked call from Kerri telling them I've had a heart attack, they are a little surprised to see that Kerri and I are laughing. I am pleased to report that my default reaction to almost everything – laughing – is unchanged by a broken heart.

The smile is soon wiped off my face though, when Young Doctor tells me I will be admitted to hospital and monitored and treated as if I have had a heart attack while tests are carried out. These tests include, but are not limited to, daily blood tests, an echocardiogram, and my favourite, the angiogram.* The angiogram is the definitive test for 'heart attack' patients, as it can tell exactly what is going on with the arteries and if the heart is diseased.

A few days later, the angiogram results confirm that my heart is not diseased, just a weird shape now, like the rest of me. My EF is 40, apparently. I have no idea what this means.**

Following all these tests, where no blockages or clots are found, takotsubo syndrome is confirmed.

I have a lot of time – six days – lying in my hospital bed to think things through. How did this happen to me?

I think back to the days after Susan died, when I went into a numbed state of shock. Having to deal with my mum's demands at the time meant that I didn't grieve for Susan properly. Susan

---

*Contrary to this statement, the angiogram is my least favourite of all of the procedures I have ever had – see page 115 to find out why.
**'EF' stands for 'ejection fraction' and is a measurement of the percentage of blood passing through the left ventricle of the heart. A normal EF is between 55 and 70%. In the event of takotsubo, EF normally returns to normal quite quickly, within 12 weeks[3] (although this is not definitive).

was a huge part of the last 10 years of my life, and was a big part of my future. We had plans. Losing her was incomprehensible, and acceptance has not yet come. I still walk around saying out loud, 'How is it possible that she's not here?'

And I think of when Mum died.

It had been March 17th, St Patrick's Day. I got the call in the morning, and that night I went out to a pre-planned gig. Not just any gig, my son's gig. That night, he played a song that Mum had been asking him to learn – *Vincent*. He never got around to learning it while she was alive, because at the time it felt like one more of her tiresome demands, but on the day she died, he did learn it. He played it that night and I broke down, inevitably.

But there are also photos of me on that same night, laughing and dancing with my friends.

Two days later I was in Seattle for a Paolo Nutini gig.

(By now you must be thinking I'm a Paolo Nutini super-fan, or stalker. It is mere coincidence that I was at one of his gigs on the day Susan died, and again two days after Mum died.)

I tucked my grief away and got on with my life. In other words, I stayed calm and carried on. It would be another seven months before I had my heart 'event'.

What actually happened here is that I squashed my emotions down like a rubbish compactor. I don't know if this was shock, or some kind of defence mechanism. Better to go to a Paolo Nutini gig than face grief head on.

In retrospect, I believe that grief is a process that needs to be worked through. You've probably never heard that before. I am a genius.

Suppressing it, pretending it's not happening, drinking or medicating through it, avoiding talking about it, about the person – none of this is healthy. It is putting an unfair burden on our minds, and of course our bodies.

(I am not saying I did all of these things, but I probably did most, if not all, of these things.)

I languish in the hospital with these thoughts tumbling around in my head, trying to make sense of it all, whilst trying to understand this new health condition that I have; one that even the doctors don't seem to be able to explain. Nobody can tell me what actually happened to me; what happened to my heart; what will happen now.

I am released from hospital after six days, following an echocardiogram and more blood tests that I never know the results of. The doctor who discharges me says this: 'Going forward, our only recommendation for you is to live a life without stress.'

A group of nurses and doctors collects at the hospital exit, laughing hysterically, rolling around on the floor clutching their stomachs whilst waving to me as I leave. 'Goodbye!' they shout through their guffawing. 'Good luck to you!'

OK, that did not happen, but it might as well have done. I am sent back into the world like a confused child, floating on a narrow brown-tinged river, in a small wooden craft, without an oar. Or in this case, a paddle.

# Chapter Ten

# A life without stress

*November 2023*
*Canada*

Going forward, the stress of trying to live a life without stress is overwhelming and actually laughably impossible. Every time I encounter so much as a driver not indicating when they exit a roundabout* I start clutching my chest and announcing I'm having 'another heart attack'. A complete over-exaggeration of course, especially as I technically did not have a heart attack in the first place.

For the first two weeks after I am released, I avoid driving altogether. When I do start driving again, I notice that when I encounter any form of aggression or arrogance on the road, or people not indicating when they exit a roundabout, I get a sharp pain in my heart. I tell this to my cardiologist at my three-week follow-up, and as he looks at me with a smirk that suggests he thinks I am a lunatic, he has no explanation for it. 'Your heart is

---

*Pet peeve alert! In our part of Canada, drivers have not been taught to use a roundabout but for some reason (as a sick joke?) the city councils have started putting them everywhere; and for some other, inexplicable, reason I am obsessed with this. It makes me so... stressed.

healthy,' he tells me. 'There is no reason for you to get a pain.' This is more than a little confusing.

I also tell him that I feel depressed, exhausted, sluggish and not at all like myself. 'What medication are you on?' he asks me. After wondering briefly why he wouldn't know this, I reply: 'Metoprolol and Apo-Perindopril.' (I don't say that, because I can't remember – or pronounce – either of those drugs, but luckily I have a photo of them on my phone.)

'Ah. What you are experiencing are side-effects from those medications,' he says.

'Right. Can I come off them then?'

'No,' he says. 'You need to give your heart time to heal.'

*But you said my heart was healthy*, I don't say.

This conversation illustrates a commonality for TTS sufferers: a *tiny* bit of uncertainty when it comes to what we are told after a takotsubo event. Depending of course on where we are in the world, there seems to be a general lack of cohesive and reliable medical information; what there is available is sometimes confusing and contradictory. In some cases, lacking altogether.

The cardiologist does say one thing that is reassuring* though. As I am leaving his office, he says, 'You're lucky... most people your age don't get a chance to check out their heart health. You

---

*When I say reassuring, I mean totally perplexing. So.... I can relax, knowing that I have free rein to eat cream cakes, drink alcohol and take up smoking if I so desire; yet also knowing that my left ventricle can puff up like a Japanese octopus trap, restricting the blood flow to my body, all because I'm driving behind someone who doesn't know how to use a roundabout?

have had a full heart check-up, and you can relax knowing your arteries are clear.'

Obviously I am confused: it is almost as if I had a heart attack, but didn't actually have a heart attack. I have been diagnosed with a condition that on the surface sounds flighty and kind of exotic, and not really a big deal, but in reality, is serious and life-altering. I have been given medication, but not really an explanation for why. The medication makes me feel worse than I feel when I am not on it. I have been given no treatment plan, no advice and no prognosis.

It is recommended that I do heart rehab, which turns out to be an online class where I am instructed how to exercise, eat healthily and keep the aspirin handy. (All great, except I know all that, and seem to have been lumped in with people who have actual heart disease. But I don't have heart disease. Do I?)

I trust the doctors and what they tell me, because – well, they are doctors. I believe it when I am told it is extremely unlikely I will have enough event; that I will recover fully; that I will feel 'normal' again very quickly; that I need certain meds; that I can exercise; that I can go back to work; that I can fly within a month, etc, etc etc.

But the problem is, the doctors who are telling me this are not takotsubo specialists. Some of them admit they have had to look up many of my questions. I am almost certain some of them have never come across the condition before. TTS seems to be on the rise. It is life-changing, and it can be fatal – so it is not to be sniffed at. We are not talking about the common cold here. Sorry, I thought it was time for a joke, even a bad one.

There are very few doctors, even those who specialise in the heart, who fully understand TTS. The general dismissiveness and lack of real knowledge I encounter are startling. This is a feeling that is not conducive to living without stress. We are not talking about a toe, or an earlobe here; we are talking about a heart! I know I said I'm not a doctor, but I do know that the heart is a fairly important organ.

There is more research into takotsubo now than 10 years ago, but you have to search to find it. I am given no literature on the condition (although much later I find out that in Canada, a leaflet is available courtesy of the University of Ottawa Heart Institute); the booklets I am given are for heart disease, not TTS.

I am grateful for my doctors, who did take it seriously, and who did keep me in hospital for six days while they carried out every test necessary, as well as a few that weren't. And I am not blaming them for the woeful lack of information, consistent advice and ability to answer questions. It's not their fault they haven't dealt with this condition much, if at all, in their careers. But the lack of true understanding is worrying.

(And also, I admit here, despite the title of my book, that when the medical professionals call it 'broken heart syndrome', this does somehow demean it, and contributes to the generally dismissive attitude, almost like it is not worthy of real investigation and research). Throw in the fact that the condition is known to affect a large percentage of post-menopausal women (80-90% of those who are diagnosed with TTS are female[4]), and we are in danger of assuming that there is some kind of 'female hysteria' leading to hearts breaking all over the place.

There are way too many people with this condition who have been short-changed with the care they receive. I have spoken to many patients who have not felt heard, cared for or taken seriously. In some cases, a blatant disregard for the condition has led to catastrophic results. At the very least, doctors should be sitting up and taking notice; educating themselves.

So, anyway, sorry – I got sidetracked there. Rant over. Back to my story.

The weeks following my release from hospital are tough. I am exhausted. I am frightened. I am unable/too scared to exercise. I feel emotionally sensitive, like I am a fragile butterfly with bruised wings, hesitant to fly again.

Speaking of flying again, I have a pre-planned trip back to the UK booked for five weeks after my event. I ask my cardiologist if it will be OK to fly; he doesn't really know and he can't very well Google it right in front of me, so he says, 'Yes'. Then he says, 'If not going will cause more stress than going, then you should go'. This is not even a tiny bit reassuring.

After much deliberation, and protests from my worried family, because actually nobody seems to know if it is OK to fly five weeks after a TTS, I decide that I feel well enough to go. I will avoid stress, I reassure them, somewhat naïvely.

My trip to England is extremely stressful. I have a Christmas tree business which is intense and demanding. Despite the long hours, physically demanding manual work and a lot of stress that any seasonal business might involve, I survive the two weeks, though I do lie awake most nights terrified that I am over-taxing my body and my mind.

In a way I am grateful that I get the chance to test my heart; if I can get through these few weeks without having another episode, then I am clearly fully recovered.

(Nobody tells me – and it is months later when I learn for myself – that the heart takes five to six months to go back to normal after a TTS event.)

While in England, one of my friends tells me that they have noticed I seem different. This forces me to look at myself and ask some questions. What exactly has changed?

What has changed, I think, is everything. My world has become smaller. I am sweating the small stuff. I am sweating the small stuff, the big stuff, the stuff I didn't even used to know was stuff. I have a new-found anxiety. My sparkle has gone. I overreact to things. Socialising has become a chore. I hate small talk. I don't much like big talk either. I worry almost constantly. I have a vulnerability that I never had before. All of these things are new to me. And I do think my mum's suicide has a part to play in this, but I am more certain that it is the TTS that has changed me as a person.

Some of the women who share their stories later in the book speak of having a renewed appreciation for life. I am more than happy for them, but I feel the opposite. I feel like something has been taken away from me. I think it is probably the assumption of health that has gone, and the freedom that comes with it.

I am not strong, after all. I am fragile. I suppose, in a way, we all are.

# Chapter Eleven

# In the aftermath

The nature of writing a book means that by the time it is published, some of the information and content will already be outdated. There will no doubt be medical and research advancements in what is known about takotsubo – and I really hope I am right about that. In the time since takotsubo made its unwelcome appearance into my world, to the time I am sending this book off to the publisher, I have noticed an increase in information available online. I encourage you to look for it.

And in fact, just as we go to print, Professor Dana Dawson has shared some exciting news: she and her team have finally been awarded funding to conduct a trial which will study the implications of medication in the long-term outcomes in takotsubo cardiomyopathy. The trial will take seven years to complete, but afterwards patients and doctors will have precise, scientifically correct treatment guidance to follow. As Professor Dawson says, 'This will put an end to the haze that currently exists regarding treatment of this condition'.

Also, results from the most recent study from InterTAK (International Registry for Takotsubo) have just been released. The study covered 3957 takotsubo patients diagnosed between

2004 and 2021. It shows, among other things, the following noteworthy updates:
- An increased number of men being diagnosed with takotsubo, up from 10% to 15%.
- An increased proportion of physical triggers, up from 39% to 58% over the period, making physical causes more common than emotional/psychological.
- A significant increase in the proportion of people dying within 60 days of diagnosis. But also a landmark analysis – excluding patients who died within the first 60 days – showed no differences in numbers of people dying within one year.[5]

In addition, there is a time lapse between my own story with takotsubo, which started in 2023, and the time you are reading this. You may wonder what, if anything, has changed for me.

As I write this, it's 18 months since my mum's suicide, and 11 months since my takotsubo attack. I am OK. Ish.

Physically, in the absence of any actual tests (I have had no follow-ups), I feel almost fully recovered. I do think that a lingering effect of TTS, for me, has been a general feeling of tiredness. I tire much more quickly than I used to and sometimes, despite eating healthily and exercising regularly, I feel generally exhausted. I have to admit that my age (almost 59 now) could be a contributory factor though. I don't really *feel* old, but I think my body does.

I have days where I feel like my body is plugged into a live socket; like my insides are fizzy and my blood is made from cola. At those times, I take deep breaths and practise mindfulness until the fizziness dissipates; until, essentially, I go flat again. I know this is caused by a mind-body connection, and I have to calm my mind to calm my body.

I have had stressful situations in the past four months – and I am still here. I can walk up the heart-thumping hill again, and I can (almost) do it without fear of having another attack. I am grateful for my healthy heart, but I will be more grateful when I have no fear at all. I want to be fearless again.

I very occasionally get a twinge in my heart – sometimes, but not always, as a result of physical or emotional stress – but I believe, after my research for this book, that this is not an indication of a potential second attack. I cannot explain what it is or why I get it, and I don't think anyone can, yet. But I am hopeful that one day, we will have the answers we crave.

My heart still feels fragile, as if I need to protect it from stress – which of-course is true, and this is stressful, because it is also impossible. I think there is a natural fear that comes from not just a sense of my own mortality, but the lack of any kind of assuredness, or at the very least information, that I would get if I had almost any other condition. It feels like all of us who have TTS are lost on a lonely highway, searching for a map to navigate to the right road, but getting no direction along the way. There is no GPS available to us; it is not yet on the market.

2023 was generally a sobering experience for me. Not so sobering that I am actually sober, though. I still drink wine, and I still eat chocolate. I want to live my life. And I believe in our doing the things that make us happy, in moderation of course.

My mental health, I would say, has not recovered as quickly as my physical health. I am a different person to the one I once was; grief and illness have changed me. I think grief changes everyone; and I am certain that takotsubo does too.

The grief I feel for my mother's passing has evolved from its initial stage of anger and blame, to punch-in-the-gut sorrow. I feel I am only now starting to process the reality of it. Now, when I see someone who resembles her (usually an eccentrically-dressed, elderly woman bounding along the street laden with shopping bags), or catch a whiff of an aroma that reminds me of her (usually cigarette smoke), I feel a pang of sadness that used to be fury. The bitterness has given way to heartache. Are the occasional twinges related? Maybe, but I don't think so.

This exclusive place I inhabit – the broken-hearted suicide-bereaved club – is a grim and lonely place to be. I really don't want anyone else in my club, for their sake. For my sake, though, I sometimes long for company; a visitor who attempts to understand the pain I endure.

I am still finding my way through it all, and I have no idea what will come out of the other side. I am hoping for a new, improved me, one who is less self-critical, one who is kinder to herself, one who is not burdened by guilt or regret; one who can live a life that Mum, and Susan, would have been proud of.

I no longer have the mindset that I don't care, because I do care. I want to be healthy, mentally and physically. When my mind starts to wander down the painful road of grief, or that crippling highway of fear, I put my foot on the brake, and tell myself to think positive thoughts. I actually say out loud, 'Think of something good!' and straight away I can change my thought pattern. Most of the time.

I know that in time I will grow to be strong again. Somatic therapy is helping me. This therapy explores how the body expresses deeply painful experiences, applying mind–body healing to aid trauma recovery. This kind of therapy seems to apply to me.

And after just four sessions, I have already had a couple of revelations. Delving into my past, learning about my sadness and loneliness as a child and teenager, is helping me to forgive myself for the patterns I have developed as an adult: seemingly controlling behaviour, impatience, intolerance – the things I regret the most in my relationship with my mother.

Through somatic therapy, I have learned a technique which I want to share with you. It is a simple one: touch your heart. If you are feeling stressed or overwhelmed, take a moment, and physically hold your hand over your heart for a few seconds.

Touching your heart has been proven to release oxytocin, the 'love hormone'. At 58 years old, I am only just learning this. You might already know it, but to me, it is revolutionary. Touching my heart has a deep and primal effect on me. I am not only experiencing the 'love hormone', and consequently feeling instantly calmer and more connected to myself, but I am honouring the very thing that is sustaining me. Yes, it is the same thing that could have killed me, but it didn't, did it? It just gave me a warning. It said, 'Sit down. Calm down'.

Actually, it said, 'SIT THE FUCK DOWN! CALM THE FUCK DOWN!'

I had no choice but to sit (and calm) the fuck down.

I deeply regret that I didn't have this therapy sooner in my life. I wish I didn't have to lose my mother to suicide, and then get a broken heart, before I sought it out. I think I could have been more tolerant of my mum if I had been more patient, more understanding.

And if *she'd* had therapy... well I believe her life, and death, would likely have been very different.

And so my journey continues, a journey in which I have to trust that my broken heart is slowly healing. In the process, I am learning to forgive my mother and to forgive myself.

I am learning to be a new me, one who is not defined by suicide, grief and octopus pots.

# PART II

# Understanding the octopus pot syndrome

# Chapter Twelve

# The fun stuff

I call it fun stuff because I want you to read this bit, so I am trying to lure you in with a blatant lie. It is not much fun, because I can't be sarcastic or flippant, but it is important. This chapter deals with facts, research and expert opinion.

## What actually is takotsubo?

We have all heard the term 'dying of a broken heart' – a term which has been, and still is, used in a kind of mythical rather than a factual way. A simple online search will uncover stories of people throughout history, including some celebrities, dying quickly after a loved one has passed, or experiencing symptoms similar to what we now know could have been takotsubo (TTS), following a traumatic event.

These experiences typically went unrecognised as TTS, as the condition was not fully identified until fairly recently.

With advances in modern medicine, several newer cardiac conditions have become easier to comprehend; TTS is one of these. However, there is a long way to go to understanding the condition, what its true causes are and how it should be treated.

Originally, as I mentioned, it was thought that TTS affected *only* post-menopausal women, and as such there appeared to be a link with a hormonal imbalance. However, as more research has been conducted, it has been found that TTS can also affect men, younger women and even children.

Men with TTS often have a physical trigger – for example, a severe illness – and tend to have worse outcomes compared to women. And of course, if a man were to experience TTS, say following an illness, or a young woman were to experience TTS following a job promotion, then 'broken heart syndrome' would be a confusing diagnosis.

Do we know anything about why takotsubo occurs in some people and not others? The simple answer to this is, no; and clearly much more research is needed.

In a review conducted in 2021, it was noted that: 'There are still many aspects of TTS that we still do not fully understand. Each of the pathophysiological hypotheses in the study were an important contribution, but in isolation, none of them fully explains all the mechanisms that lead to TTS.'[6]

We know that a large percentage of patients are female. But males also get it.

We know that the majority of sufferers are middle-aged. But children and young adults have been known to get it. We know that physical or emotional stress, or sometimes a happy event, can cause it. But we also know that sometimes there are no triggers at all.

There are suggestions that TTS is caused after stress hormones are released into the bloodstream as a reaction to those triggers.

But this doesn't explain why someone who is experiencing absolutely no stress – physical, mental, or otherwise – someone who is, for instance, sitting on their sofa watching TV – can suddenly and confusingly find themselves being diagnosed with 'broken heart syndrome'.

The cause of takotsubo remains a 'scientific mystery' – these words are taken directly from the British Heart Foundation website.

## What happens to the heart in TTS?

The left ventricle of the heart has the largest muscle mass of all the heart's chambers and, in a normal heart, it contracts strongly and uniformly to enable it to pump blood to the rest of the body, where it is needed. When TTS occurs, it mainly affects the left ventricle and impairs its ability to pump properly. The wall of the ventricle becomes weakened and it takes on an abnormal shape. This, in turn, reduces the efficiency of the ventricle.

While it is principally the left ventrical, the right ventricle has also been known to be affected.[6]

## Ejection fraction (EF)

'Left ventricular ejection fraction' (EF) refers to the percentage of blood ejected from the left ventricle with each heartbeat. Some experts say that an EF of 50% is normal, although others consider an EF of 50-55% as being borderline. The left ventricle does not empty completely, and so the upper level of normal for EF is considered to be around 70-75%.

In the first stages of TTS, the EF can be as low as 20%, though this varies in each case. When the EF is low, it can cause shortness of breath as blood accumulates in the left ventricle.

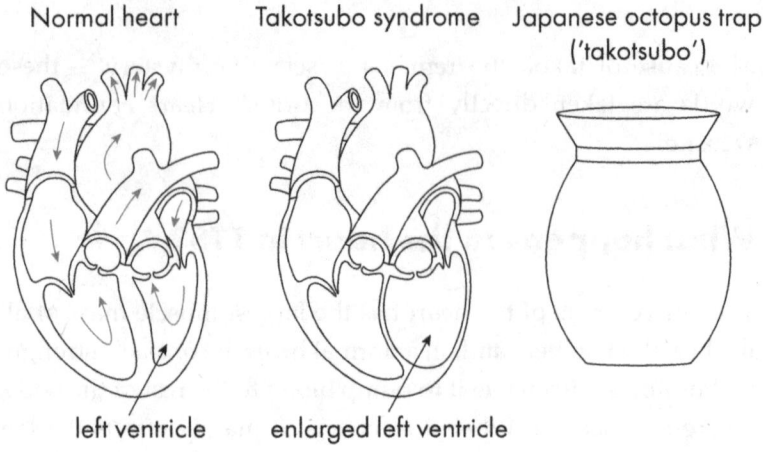

## Catecholamines and takotsubo syndrome

Catecholamines, such as dopamine and adrenaline, are hormones that the brain, nerve tissues and adrenal glands produce. People who develop TTS are usually found to have high levels of catecholamines. When a person experiences physical or emotional stress, catecholamines are released into the bloodstream and they have effects on the body that prepare us for the fight or flight response.

Some typical effects of catecholamines are increased heart rate, blood pressure and blood glucose levels, as well as epinephrine (also known as adrenalin).

## How do you mend a broken heart?*

*Confusing title alert! If all TTS patients had a 'broken heart' – if their condition was caused by something which might be considered heartbreaking – then the long-term treatment plan might be a little easier to devise (though I can't for the life of me think what it might be, other than stress management: rest, de-stress, relax etc...). As it is, there is no definitive treatment plan for TTS sufferers, and the fact that there is no recognised cause of the condition could, of course, be one of the reasons for that.

What about the people who have ongoing and long-term effects from the condition? What about those with other health conditions? What about those whose TTS was not caused by a stress event? Those people don't have answers yet.

There is clearly still so much to learn and research to be done on this. As I am not a doctor, I am certainly not qualified to give advice here on how to recover from it. Actually, even if I was a doctor, I probably still couldn't give you any advice on how to recover from it. There is still so little known about treatment and recovery. But I have done some research, and have spoken to some experts, and so below I have some guidelines which hopefully go some way to helping if you have experienced something similar to me.

## Ideas and suggestions to aid recovery from takotsubo

### *Do your research*

Join a Facebook group. I got more answers from Facebook groups than I did from any doctor. Talk to other people who have experienced TTS. In the Facebook group set up by Caron

Curragh (who contributed the Foreword), you will not only find other people who have experienced TTS, and who can offer guidance and support, but also a wealth of useful information in the 'files' section, pointing you towards the most recent studies.

The internet generally will, of course, provide you with a host of information. This website, run in conjunction with the Facebook group, is highly recommended: www.takotsubo.net

**Exercise**
Immediately following the event, the single most important thing to do is to rest until you feel able to resume normal activity level. Start slowly and listen to your body. But when you're ready, you can start to bring exercise back into your life. Easy does it.

**Walking**
Before TTS, I could undertake a strenuous and long hike pretty easily. After my TTS, I was terrified to even walk up a flight of stairs; and when I did, I felt weak and tearful. After 10 days of pure rest, I was desperate to get back to walking. I started with a tentative 10 minutes a day on the flat, slowly increasing the time and intensity each day.

During these walks I often felt breathless and fearful, but once I had my confidence back, I realised that I was putting restrictions on myself rather than listening to my body. I am now back to an hour a day, incorporating hills. I use this time to listen to music or podcasts, but also as a kind of think-tank. My best problem-solving is done when I am walking. Walking is, in my opinion, the best exercise of all. Safe, free and therapeutic, walking gives you a boost of serotonin as well as an essential dose of vitamin D.

But of course this is different for everyone. I feel that anxiety and depression can interfere in this process. For me, I needed to overcome the fear I had, but once I knew my heart could cope with it, I was soon back to walking confidently.

## Swimming

Over 20 years ago, when I lived in England and was in my 30s, I suffered with night-time panic attacks. They came on in the dead of night, with no warning, and took over my whole body. I would go into a state of disassociation; it was terrifying. I eventually went to talk to my GP, a young, progressive doctor who got out her prescription pad and prescribed... swimming. I was given three swimming sessions a week for six months, paid for by the NHS. The panic attacks went away and never came back.

As a result, I am a big fan of swimming, for both physical and mental health. It has so many benefits: it is invigorating, meditative and obviously physically beneficial.

## Yoga

I also am a big fan of yoga, as you know. Am I in danger of becoming a yoga bore? Don't answer that please. I took up yoga when I was in my fifties, and I get anxious when I go more than two days without it. My almost-daily practice did not save me from having the TTS, but it has helped me ground myself in the aftermath.

Yoga is beneficial to our mental as well as physical health and has been proven to reduce stress. It encourages us to relax, slow our breathing and focus on the present, shifting the balance from the sympathetic nervous system and the flight-or-fight response to the parasympathetic system and the relaxation response.

Hatha yoga, especially, is a good stress reliever because of its slower pace and easier movements.

**Yoga nidra**

Yoga nidra is also an amazing tool for resetting the nervous system and for healing from trauma. I have used it in the past as a sleep aid, but since having takotsubo, I now know it can benefit the somatic system as well.

## *Take a bath!*

Take an Epsom salt bath. Epsom salts extract toxins at the skin level, help your body to absorb magnesium, and generally promote relaxation. Top tip: add a cup of baking soda to help detox and exfoliate – this helps address inflammation and promotes sleep.

## *Practise cyclic sighing*

This is a method that is used to help lower stress and anxiety levels, particularly during negotiations, conflict or difficult conversations. It is particularly useful if you get a shock or a fright, helping to work through the shock and expel the emotions.

Method:
- Breathe in through your nose.
- When you have comfortably filled your lungs, take another, deeper sip of air to expand your lungs as much as possible.
- Then, very slowly, exhale through your mouth until all the air is gone.
- Repeat the cycle for around 5 minutes.

## *Practise breath work*

Deep breathing is known to be a stress reliever. You can do it anywhere. You are already halfway there, actually, as you are breathing right now. Please do some research; there are books,

YouTube videos and websites that give lots of information on breathing techniques. You could also find an in-person class where you can practise deep breathing in a controlled environment.

## *Practise meditation*

Meditation encourages us to quieten the stream of jumbled thoughts that can crowd our minds and cause stress. It provides a sense of calm, peace and balance that promotes emotional wellbeing and overall health.

You can practise guided meditation, guided imagery, mindfulness, visualisation and other forms of meditation anywhere at any time. There are a multitude of apps, books and YouTube videos available to help.

## *Avoid unhealthy habits*

For some of us it is easy to turn to unhealthy habits when we are stressed: abuse of alcohol or illegal substances; over-eating, and smoking to name a few. Even drinking too much caffeine can be detrimental to our health. These habits often increase rather than decrease our stress levels. Best to avoid them.*

## *Laugh!*

I am a strong believer in humour. One of my favourite things to do is to laugh. There are studies showing that laughing can have a positive impact on mental health, anxiety and stress.[7] Laughing releases dopamine; it also causes positive changes in the body, and cools our stress responses.

*Hypocrite alert! As I have mentioned, I do drink wine – but no longer to excess.

Watch or read something funny, read some jokes, tell jokes or surround yourself with upbeat friends and family, the ones who make you laugh. Or give laughing yoga a try. I have tried this (because why not?) and, believe me, it is hilarious.

## Connect with other people

It is, I feel, a natural reaction to want to isolate yourself after a TTS event, or when you are generally stressed. You feel vulnerable, scared and sad. But, by isolating, you are perpetuating any feelings of despondency, and this, of course, can lead to a sense of loneliness and sometimes hopelessness.

Try to reach out to your family and friends – one good friend who listens can make a difference. Or make new social connections.

So take a coffee break with a friend or acquaintance; email, call or text a relative; or visit your place of worship. In time, you might want to consider volunteering for a charity – in other words, help yourself while helping others.

## Make yourself a priority

You might be impatient to get back to 'normal', but it is imperative that you listen to your body. Learn to say no, learn to delegate, learn to set boundaries. Putting yourself first, not second, will lessen stress, anger and resentment.

## Get enough sleep

Stress can cause us to have trouble falling asleep. When we have too much to do and too much to think about, our sleep invariably suffers. But sleep is essential to our wellbeing and recovery; it is the time when our bodies and brains recharge.

How well and how long we sleep can affect our mood, energy level, focus and overall functioning.

If you have trouble sleeping, make sure that you have a quiet, relaxing bedtime routine: put phones and tablets out of reach; ensure the area you sleep in is cool, dark and quiet; and try to stick to a regular schedule. Don't eat a big meal or drink alcohol before bed.

Instead of watching TV or looking at your phone, listen to soothing music, meditate or practise Yoga nidra.

## *Keep a journal*

Writing down your thoughts and feelings can be a good release for otherwise pent-up emotions. Don't think about what to write — let it flow. Use a notebook, journal or computer. No one else needs to read it.

Once you're finished, you can throw it away or delete it if you want to; or not.

## *Take up a hobby*

Keeping ourselves busy with a hobby keeps us focused on what we are doing rather than what we think we should be doing. Playing or listening to music is a good stress reliever. It can provide a mental distraction, lessen muscle tension and lower stress hormones. Turn up the volume and let your mind be absorbed by the melodies.

If music isn't your thing, indulge in another hobby that you love

– reading, drawing, colouring – or take up a new one. How about gardening? Knitting? Painting?

Or join a club. How about singing in a choir? Creative writing? Bridge club? A walking group would be perfect.

### Seek counselling

For me, it took a takotsubo event to realise that I probably needed some kind of therapy. (This is where you say, 'Duh!'.)

As Professor Dana Dawon tells us on page 107, there are studies underway into CBT (cognitive behavioural therapy) and its benefits for the ongoing recovery of TTS patients. I believe that CBT will be shown to be very beneficial, and I for one will be exploring it at some point.

For now, I have chosen somatic therapy because it is relevant to my experience.

But of course, each of our journeys and needs are different and individual. I encourage you to explore what is out there, if therapy or counselling is what you feel you need. Professional counsellors or therapists can help you find the sources of your stress and learn new coping tools.

'What is somatic therapy?' you might ask. Kerri Neild, a relational somatic therapist based in BC, Canada, says: 'Soma is a Greek word for unity of body and mind. Somatic therapy combines the right-brain experience of embodiment, empathy and intuition with the left-brain experience of knowledge and meaning. Relational somatic therapy includes the body in the present moment experience to help resolve the emotional reaction of past trauma and to regulate current experiences of pain, adversity or joy in relationship.'

Somatic therapy can help with trauma, PTSD, anxiety and depression, chronic pain and stress management.

## *Implement dietary and lifestyle changes*

Whilst takotsubo is not linked to poor diet (as far as it's known), it is always a good idea to implement healthy eating habits, and for that reason, in Chapter 16, you will find some heart-healthy recipes and suggestions. In the meantime, here are some tips for making immediate changes to your diet and lifestyle.
- Eat regular meals throughout the day.
- Eat your first meal within 1 to 2 hours of waking.
- Increase your intake of healthy fats – for example, avocado, unsalted nuts and seeds, and nut butters
- Increase your fibre intake: fibre is found in fruit and vegetables, whole grains, nuts, seeds and legumes (like kidney beans, chickpeas and lentils).
- Use olive or avocado oil for cooking and salad dressings.
- Reduce your intake of red meat.
- Choose lower-fat dairy products and milk alternatives.
- Eliminate or reduce processed foods.
- Stay away from deep-fried foods, pre-packaged snack foods and commercial baked goods.
- Choose brightly coloured fruit and veg and generally increase your intake. Eat them raw, roasted, steamed or stir fried.
- Choose orange and dark green vegetables more often: carrots, butternut squash, sweet potatoes, romaine lettuce, broccoli and kale
- Choose whole fruits over juice.
- Aim to fill half your plate with veg and/or fruit, a quarter with protein and a quarter with whole grains

- Choose whole grains such as whole wheat, oatmeal, bran, quinoa, wild rice. Avoid white flour, white bread and white pasta.
- Add legumes to your diet – for instance, lentils, kidney beans and chickpeas
- Eat more fish – particularly fatty fish. Aim for two servings per week.
- Increase your water intake.
- Use less sugar in your meal preparation.
- Use less salt – replace salt with seasonings: herbs, spices, lemon juice, garlic, vinegars.
- Limit take-aways and restaurant foods.
- Limit alcohol consumption.
- Eliminate smoking and tobacco products.
- Consider taking supplements – talk to a health practitioner and/or your GP about what is right for you.
- If you are female, please educate yourself on the menopause, peri-menopause, hormones and their effects on our heart, organs and the body in general. I recommend this website: www.thepauselife.com, which was set up by menopause expert Dr Mary Claire Haver.

# Chapter Thirteen

# Expert opinions on takotsubo

To find out more about takotsubo, I talked to two leading UK cardiologists: Dr Sanjay Gupta, based in York, and Professor Dana Dawson, based in Aberdeen.

## Dr Sanjay Gupta

Dr Sanjay Gupta is a consultant cardiologist/heart specialist at York Teaching Hospital in the UK. His YouTube channel can be found here: https://www.youtube.com/user/YorkCardiology.

**Have you encountered many cases of takotsubo in your 29-year career?**

*Absolutely. We see it quite a lot. In fact, I think it's on the increase.*

**Can you explain the difference between takotsubo and a traditional heart attack?**

*What we call a 'heart attack' is a consequence of diseased arteries. Not enough blood can reach the heart muscle. But when the heart arteries are clear – when there are no blockages – then we say, OK this could be takotsubo. The possibility of that diagnosis starts to be entertained once the angiogram has been done and it has demonstrated clean arteries; then it's absolutely confirmed for certain after a period of time has elapsed, usually two to three months, when the heart is re-scanned and we can see that the weakness in the heart has gone away.*

**How can you be sure that a patient has suffered a takotsubo episode rather than a heart attack?**

*When the patient comes in, it's very difficult to be absolutely confident that it's one and not the other. Takotsubo is actually a diagnosis that is made with the benefit of hindsight; more often than not, when a patient is admitted, they have signs and symptoms that suggest they have had a heart attack, and at that point it would be presumptuous to put these down to takotsubo, because the difference between a traditional heart attack and takotsubo is that the damage that is seen initially is reversible, while it is permanent in patients who have had a heart attack. So what you have to do when the patient first comes in is an angiogram. Then when the angiogram shows normal coronary arteries, we can start really entertaining the takotsubo diagnosis. The question then is, how can we be certain? Well, a heart attack will cause permanent death of the heart muscle, whereas takotsubo does not. In takotsubo, you don't have the death of any tissue; you have a punch-drunk state. So the heart doesn't move because the cells are punch-drunk. They are stunned, not dead.*

**What tests in the early stages are useful in determining the difference between a heart attack and takotsubo?**

*At a very minimum, when you go into A&E with chest pain, you would expect at least an ECG and a troponin blood* test. If the level of troponin is elevated, that tells you there is some damage to the heart. And then you would have an echocardiogram, which would possibly show the changed shape of the heart.

An MRI can also be done, when a dye called gadolinium is injected, which accumulates in dead tissue. So typically, in a heart attack, you will see some dead tissue due to the deposition of gadolinium in the scarred areas. In contrast, in takotsubo, you will not see deposits of gadolinium, and that tells you there is no scarring, which means that that tissue is still living, even though it is not contributing to movement at this stage.

**What is the significance of troponin?**

Elevated troponin in the blood tells you there has been damage to the heart. It will go up in a heart attack, and it will go up in takotsubo. When the troponin level is elevated, it tells you two things: one, there is something going on with the heart; and two, that if you do not do anything about this, there is an increased risk of something catastrophic happening in the next 14 days. This means troponin is very helpful because it points to the diagnosis, but it also tells you a little bit about prognosis and what is going to happen in the future.

**Do you have any insight into why some people would die from takotsubo while others recover quickly, as I did? Could an underlying condition contribute to death from this condition?**

No. When you have a heart attack, you damage a significant part of the heart and less blood is pumped around the body. When you have a takotsubo episode, the same thing happens. It is just that with takotsubo, the function of the heart gets better over a period of time. In the acute phase, however, it is still a weak heart.

*You need time for the heart to recover from takotsubo; whilst it is weak, it can still misbehave like an ordinary heart attack will.*

**So that's why it's important to deal with takotsubo as soon as possible?**

*Absolutely. You need to be in a monitored setting. As long as the heart is very weak, it needs supporting.*

**Can you explain why TTS does not show up in a post mortem?**

*In a post mortem, the heart is no longer working. The only thing which tells us the heart is malfunctioning is it's not moving, but because when you're dead, the heart's not moving anyway, a reduction in movement can't be seen; all we can look for is evidence of scarring. And in takotsubo, there is no dead tissue and no scarring, so therefore, no, it won't show up on a post-mortem examination.*

**What happens physiologically when the ventricle enlarges?**

*The heart is a bag – a container. The only way this container gets bigger is if it contains more blood. As the heart becomes stunned and changes shape, less blood is ejected, so more blood builds up within it. When less blood is ejected, the kidneys receive less blood. This tells the body that the person is dehydrated, so they retain more water from the urine, as they would when they are truly dehydrated. This increases the volume of blood, so more blood fills the heart up. But the problem is that this person was never short of blood; the heart just wasn't strong enough to pump the blood out.*

*The heart is strained. It stretches, starts getting bigger and bigger, and the kidneys are still getting less blood. So, that's why we see this progressive enlargement, and that is why takotsubo patients are given a diuretic and an ACE inhibitor, because these are medications that tell the kidneys not to absorb water, and to let them urinate out the extra bit.*

**So, as a cardiologist, how would you attempt to explain to a takotsubo patient why they have had it?**

*All the research journals say it's a stress-induced cardiomyopathy [disease of the heart muscle]. But actually, I have spoken to lots of takotsubo patients, and many say it was just a normal day; that they were not particularly stressed. We all go through stress. Why do some people get this and not others? I would say that there must be some kind of genetic vulnerability in some people, because how many people go through divorces? How many people go through earthquakes? Or grief? Not everyone gets takotsubo. But ultimately we still don't really know what causes it.*

**Do you foresee a study being conducted into what causes takotsubo?**

*There's no way of doing that study because the first time you meet the patient is after it's happened.*

**What is the most accurate way to determine that a patient has fully recovered from takotsubo?**

*We are limited by our technology. The commonly used mechanism of assessing whether the heart is weak or not is an echocardiogram, and that's a two-dimensional modality. But the heart is not a two-dimensional structure; it's a three-dimensional structure. The heart doesn't move only in one direction; it moves in three or four; it moves vertically; it moves horizontally; it twists. So what we have done is we've taken an echocardiogram and made some crude measurements, and when those crude measurements improve, we say 'Your heart function has normalised'. But we are studying the heart at rest; we're not studying it at times of stress. So it's important to realise for everyone that what the patient tells us is more important than just us doctors looking at the scan. And that is why there is this discrepancy between patients saying, 'The doctor tells me my heart has gone back to normal', but also asking, 'Why am I so tired? Why am I not quite right?'*

*The weakness disappears on our imaging modalities after two or three months, but if you talk to patients, they'll feel symptomatic, even at two years sometimes. Professor Dawson [interviewed next] did a study where she got people to exercise and do stress testing as another way of assessing their functional status and found that there were subtle abnormalities in these patients even after up to 21 months, whereas their two-dimensional echo parameters had normalised. And that's where patients really struggle, because they say, 'I don't feel right'.*

*I think the problem is that the medical profession has kind of lost its humility; as a profession we think we know everything, and anything we don't know isn't worth knowing about. And if the patient says something which is against what we know, then the patient is mad or stressed. And this is one of the fundamental problems, because actually the only way we are going to learn is by listening to the patients.*

*If the patient is saying, 'I am still not right' two years down the line, then we shouldn't automatically just say, 'Oh, they're anxious'; we should say, 'Our imaging isn't good enough'; 'Maybe our knowledge isn't deep enough to understand everything about this condition'.*

## Is it possible to screen for and can a second TTS episode be avoided?

> The answer to both of those questions is, not really. There may be a way of screening for takotsubo if you've already had an episode, because you've already sort of highlighted yourself as someone who has that vulnerability. So, what we could potentially then do is say, let me study your genes, see if there's some kind of weird genetic makeup here, and then we can screen your children. That hasn't happened as yet, but that may be a possibility in the future.
>
> But even if you have the genetic vulnerability, that doesn't necessarily mean you will have a takotsubo episode. I don't think it's possible to screen for it.
>
> So, if an episode has caused some damage, you would be treated with medications that help to strengthen the heart. And a lot of people are now beginning to say, if that is the case, then just keep the medications going for life. We know that there are medications which are helpful when you have a weak heart.
>
> There are definitely medications which are helpful in terms of slowing the heart, reducing the likelihood of heart rhythm disturbances happening, breaking that negative feedback between the heart and the kidneys, etc. Does that mean that if you take these medications for the rest of your life, it will definitively reduce the risk of another episode happening? The problem is that we don't know. If you take the medications and don't have another episode, how do you know that the medications have prevented another episode from happening or not? You don't know, because the number of people who have a second episode is generally going to be much smaller anyway. So it's a very difficult study to do.

*And, other than medications, ongoing treatment is difficult to prescribe?*

Busy clinicians will say, 'Oh, the heart has normalised; the patient can go now; there's nothing dangerous going on anymore,' because we associate danger with the heart looking weak. So these patients then just leave; they're discharged because there's nothing else to do at that point, and therefore they get forgotten in that way.

We need more research from people like Professor Dawson and Dr Lyon. Professor Dawson's research is fascinating, where she has actually demonstrated that these people still are left with residual subtle deficiencies even though what we look for appears to have normalised.

Perhaps we could also look at genetics and say, 'Are these people genetically vulnerable?' So then we can take away this stress issue. Maybe then what we could say is, if you are genetically vulnerable, should we be giving you medications or should we be treating stress more aggressively?

*Bruce H Lipton, PhD, cellular biologist and leading voice in the field of epigenetics, writes in his book* **The Biology of Belief***: 'The results of animal studies point to the role that chronic stress plays in the creation of histamine and in the onset and promotion of cardiovascular disease. Histamine is a stress-related hormone that prepares the body to deal with anticipated injuries and inflammation when the fight-or-flight response is activated by a perceived stressor.' If that is the case, do you think histamine could possibly play a role in developing takotsubo?*

There are lots of people who go through tons of stress and nothing bad happens to them. I think that there is so much about genetic vulnerabilities that we don't understand. For example, why doesn't everyone with COVID get long COVID? Why do only 10% of people get it? There must be something about those 10% that makes them more vulnerable to long COVID.

**If his hypothesis is correct, though, would anti-histamine be a drug that could be given to TTS patients?**

The problem with all these things is that, whilst they're interesting hypotheses, the proof is not going to be in a study which shows, say, there's less inflammation in the heart if people take an anti-histamine, but in a study that takes 10,000 people, gives them a particular medication, follows them up for 50 years and sees how many have had heart attacks or have died compared with a group that didn't have the medication – that's the only way you would know.

**Are you in favour of natural supplements to help with heart health?**

I am all for exploring those ideas. But ultimately, what you want to do is get the hard outcomes that patients care about and they are only interested in two things: they want to live a long time and they want to have a good quality of life; those are the only two outcomes that truly matter.

Say you bought a car for your child and the car doesn't have a seat belt, so you are approached by two seat-belt manufacturers who say, 'Do you want to buy our seat belt for your car?' And one says, 'Our seat belt is synthetic; made in China using child labour'. And the other says, 'Our seat belt is eco-friendly. It's made only of natural products and manufactured in the most beautiful, harmonious environment. And it's cheaper than the other seat belt.' Which *seat belt do you buy? You would go for the one that has been shown to prevent death in a car accident!*

*Everything is an industry. The supplement industry; the organic food industry; everyone's trying to sell something. What you have to do is ask, 'How convinced am I that this will do the job?' The problem is you will never know whether something is extending your life, because you can only measure something after it's over.*

*The problem therefore is that when people say, 'Take this and you'll live longer,' you will never know if it has made a difference. And therefore you have to rely on data. You have to say, 'Did we measure the length of life of so many people who were a bit like me, and what did that data show? Did these people live longer?' That's how you have to evaluate the evidence.*

*Quality of life is a completely different thing. You don't need any data for that. You can say, 'When I take magnesium, I sleep better, I feel better'; then, great, take it. That is the important thing here.*

**So, that answers my question about vitamin C. Because, basically you're saying, yes, take vitamin C, but you're not going to be able to ever quantify how that has affected your quality of life or your length of life?**

*Absolutely. You can't know unless someone produces a study and says, I gave 10,000 people vitamin C, and look, they're all alive and happy and well 20 years down the line, and the group that didn't get vitamin C are all dead.*

***Some GPs have never heard of takotsubo. Do you think it's something that the medical field generally needs to address or educate doctors on?***

Yes. The Department of Health is basically producing more and more people just to do their job. Not do the job well, but just get people in and out. And so training has been curtailed. GPs and other doctors don't get the training that they used to.

I think there is a lot of scope for education. But again, the problem with all these things is that everyone is too busy. And now everyone is practising conveyor-belt medicine, or consulting Dr Google.

The reality is, you will know your body better than anyone else. And if we as doctors spend enough time talking to you, you will give us the answers. You will say things like, 'When I have a cold shower, I feel so much better'. And the doctor might then say, 'That's rubbish; that's placebo'. Well, you are saying it makes you feel better. And we should then be saying, 'That's interesting. Maybe I could ask my next patient with this condition whether they feel better too'. And that's how we can build that experience, that knowledge base.

***Do you think diet plays any role in takotsubo?***

We don't know is the answer. It's such an under-researched field. Because again, when you're trying to do a study on diet, it'll take so many people. And it'll take so long to study the effects of dietary influence on length of life. I guess it's just a case of trying to be your healthiest. Avoidance of processed foods, avoidance of sugar and alcohol, along with stress management, good sleep, regular exercise. Those are just *good lifestyle choices that everyone should be doing. The nice thing about that is they may make us live longer, but they also definitely improve our quality of life.*

## Professor Dana Dawson

Professor Dawson qualified in medicine at the University of Medicine 'Grigore T. Popa', Iasi, Romania. After completing her MRCP with the Royal College of Physicians in London and PhD in Cardiovascular Medicine at Merton College, University of Oxford, she trained in Cardiovascular Medicine in Edinburgh, Oxford and London in the UK and at the University of Virginia, Charlottesville, in the USA. In 2010 she moved to the University of Aberdeen and Aberdeen Royal Infirmary where she currently is Professor of Cardiovascular Medicine and Consultant Cardiologist.

She has made a significant contribution to advancing knowledge about acute stress-induced (takotsubo) cardiomyopathy, having delivered several landmark mechanistic clinical trials. Takotsubo studies are ongoing in Aberdeen, which leads the Scottish Takotsubo Registry that has been accruing all cases since 2010.

Professor Dawson leads the Cardiology and Cardiovascular Research Unit that has strong collaborative links with many other UK centres, participating in multi-centre clinical research studies. Here I interview her about what is known to date about takotsubo.

**Being involved in the research of this condition, is it frustrating or fulfilling?**

*From a scientific perspective it is fulfilling. Studying a medical condition which the whole world had seen for hundreds of years and not realised they were looking at is actually a privilege. The more we dig into what happens in this condition, the more fascinating it becomes. But it is also frustrating because when I am on call and patients ask: 'Why me? Why has this happened? What is the treatment? Am I going to have another one?' the answer to all of this is: 'I do not know'.*

**Do you think that in the span of your career, you will know the answers to these questions?**

*We will know more. We are able to look into investigations which we were not even dreaming of 10 years ago. Whether we will know it all, I doubt.*

**So are we any closer to knowing the answer to the question, 'Why me?'**

*We have some inklings, but we cannot answer these questions yet in the most definitive way. When we see patients with myocardial infarction, for which we know the risk factors very well, patients do not even ask 'Why me?' and they are the first to say, 'I am going to change my lifestyle'. Whereas takotsubo occurs quite out of the blue, predominantly in individuals who are otherwise by-and-large healthy. It is common to see patients who have no previous medical conditions. But we have other pointers, as we know there can be triggers to a takotsubo episode. This is what we call a 'psychosomatic interaction', in this case to exposure to any type of stressor. Any stress or physical illness can be a trigger: an asthma attack, a diabetic hypo, breaking a leg, being in a road traffic accident. These are physical changes or physical triggers. Imagine an asthma attack – one must be a bit worried experiencing it, as well as distressed because of the inability to breathe normally. So there is probably an element of both the physical illness and the shock of experiencing it. People can also have a very strong reaction to an upset, or even to happiness. There were people who developed takotsubo during weddings. On the other hand, there are people who cannot pinpoint a trigger at all.*

*From the experience of those in whom we have identified a possible trigger, we have concluded that this is likely a psychosomatic interaction. There are a few described in medicine. However, the simplest example of this is blushing – obviously not a medical condition. When you hear something that embarrasses you, you blush. You cannot control that. And some people are more likely to do that than others.*

*There are people who have a certain autoimmune condition (called cataplexy) where, if they break into powerful laughter, they lose control of their limbs and fall, having a complete inability to move for about 30 minutes, after which it spontaneously resolves. These phenomena exist and seem very bizarre, because we cannot explain them that well.*

**Have you seen any takotsubo events that are caused by alcohol consumption or diet?**

*Alcohol, yes, but only in excess. And interestingly enough, the cases of excess alcohol and takotsubo that we have seen were in men. I do not think there has been anything related to diet. We have certainly not come across that, but of course we only see a fraction of people.*

**Regarding the likelihood of having a second event, have you come across many people who have had second, or multiple, events?**

*Yes, we have seen recurrences. The 'record' was a lady who developed it eight times in the span of 40 years, and each time it was because of a different precipitating event. We do not know why some people develop it again. Most people only have one episode. We have recently published the Scottish Takotsubo Registry in which we noticed recurrences were only 8-10% – which is less than previously reported.*

**Can you tell us more about your latest study on physical exercise and mental wellbeing rehabilitation?**

*Yes, we recently looked at the impact of physical exercise on the recovery of the heart in one study and on the recovery of the brain in another study, both after the acute event. We are currently analyzing the results. We also implemented a programme for cognitive behavioural therapy (CBT) immediately after the acute index event. This was designed specifically by a consultant psychiatrist who is also an expert in psychology. Participants absolutely loved the sessions of CBT.*

**Based on the fact that I personally received no actual treatment for takotsubo, if I were to have a second event, why would I go to a hospital?**

*It is very important to go to hospital immediately. I cannot emphasise that enough. This is because the risk of any acute complication is within the first 48 hours of developing the condition.*

**Occasionally I get a little stabbing pain in my heart. And one lady in my Facebook group wondered whether this could happen because the heart has a kind of memory of the event? How common are ongoing issues such as these?**

*Often, I get a lot of inspiration from the people that we speak to, and this is a really nice way of putting it: 'memory pain'. We know that some people remain symptomatic to a certain extent afterwards. Some people remain symptomatic indefinitely. The symptoms that people seem to have are never of the same magnitude as the acute event, obviously.*

*Sometimes people experience ongoing tiredness, and that fatigue tends to persist after the acute event for some time. However, these ongoing issues – in regards to palpitations and fleeting chest pains – are not harbingers of a recurrence.*

**Your research has found that the medication they put TTS patients on, as a matter of course, is not particularly effective in takotsubo?**

*Yes, that is what we found and this comes from registry data. In a registry, there is a confounding bias as various doctors may treat patients very differently in the absence of firm evidence or guidelines. This would have to be assessed in the context of a properly designed trial in order to be able to definitively say what medication is helpful or not helpful.*

**My cardiologist could not give me a reason for why I was on the medications they put me on. Is that a common problem?**

*I think that there is genuine lack of knowledge regarding effective treatment after takotsubo. However, I think we have come a long way from 15-20 years ago when the condition was barely recognised.*

**In which case the people who are experiencing it now are quite lucky to not have been experiencing it 15 or 20 years ago?**

*Yes. Previously it would have either been dismissed or branded as a heart attack. Prior to this time, patients were misdiagnosed.*

***What is your opinion about the label 'broken heart syndrome'?***

*I know there are a lot of patients who do not like this name and I think that is because of the spin that media have put on it. The media like sensationalism. On the other hand, I think we have to recognise the fact that it has also helped in the sense of increasing awareness. Something I find fascinating is the expression 'you broke my heart' or 'I'm broken hearted'; these expressions existed way before this condition was recognised in medical circles. So I think that people knew about this before doctors defined it as a medical diagnosis.*

***If a patient died of takotsubo, but their heart went back to normal before a post mortem was carried out, how could it be determined that they had died from it?***

*This condition cannot be diagnosed on post-mortem examination to the best of our current knowledge.*

*In 2014-2015, we came across a few people who had died of this condition, and at that time I did ask the families if we could have permission to retain the heart and to examine it closely. That led us to one of the hypotheses of our studies. We noticed that there were inflammatory cells in the heart. At that stage we did not really understand if these inflammatory cells were present only in people who were unfortunate enough to die of the condition, or whether these inflammatory cells existed in everybody who experienced this condition and might be a characteristic of it. Through our investigation, we found that the inflammatory cells were there in everyone to begin with, when they experienced broken heart syndrome, and later they dissipated. So this is an inflammatory reaction that typically takes approximately six months to resolve.*

*Do you think if this was more a male-dominated condition there would be more funding available for research?*

I think the short answer is, no. One thing we found with takotsubo was that women were extremely interested to find out why this happened to them and why it occurred mostly in women. For the first time we have a clear, distinct condition in cardiovascular medicine that affects predominantly women. This is a unique opportunity to bring women to the forefront of scientific clinical research.

*If more women than men are coming forward in takotsubo studies, is there a possibility that more men have it than we know about?*

Possibly, yes. And one characteristic of the male phenotype in takotsubo is that the clinical syndrome is more severe than in women. Men also have a much higher likelihood of adverse outcomes compared to women.

*What single piece of advice would you give a newly diagnosed person? And also one who still has unresolved symptoms at six months?*

Two things: manage their expectations and take it easy through the recovery steps. The advice that your heart goes back to normal and you can go back to doing whatever you want from a few days after hospital discharge is outdated. People need to learn to pace themselves through the recovery because the heart muscle is still swollen, and we know that it remains swollen for a period of time afterwards – probably about five to six months. It is like a muscle bruise; while you have got the bruise, that muscle will still hurt, so you have to be patient and wait for all that to heal itself.

*I was discharged with an 'on your way, you're fine now…'*

> That is quite common unfortunately, but perceptions are changing and knowledge is evolving.

*What about somebody who's still got symptoms at six months or still got ongoing problems at six months?*

> So that is a little bit more difficult to answer because we do not know ourselves, to be quite honest.

*Do we as takotsubo patients have to avoid adrenaline-inducing sports or situations?*

> I think it is more complicated than just adrenaline. This is a concept that was first put forward – that a rush of endogenous, self-made adrenaline under circumstances of stress, is affecting the heart. I think this is extremely simplistic. It does not explain it at all in people who do not have a recognised stress or trigger event, which, according to some registries is up to a third. And the converse is also true: in an intensive care unit, every patient is maintained on quite high doses of adrenaline, and yet we do not see them develop takotsubo in excessive numbers.

*Having takotsubo would not be a reason to avoid something that would give you an adrenaline rush then? Say ziplining?*

> I do not think that ziplining will directly provoke this.

*What about cold-water swimming?*

> Cold can cause a very profound vagal reaction in the body. The heart rate will slow. So that is not an adrenaline reaction; it is quite the opposite. I am not sure if cold-water swimming would be advisable or not – I cannot say.

***We can't really say we should avoid anything because anything could cause it?***

*Yes, and the best evidence we have for that is the knowledge we have from recurrent cases. They are never caused by the same stressor as the initial episode.*

***Do you suspect any link to the vaccine?***

*Not as such. Not more than in any other circumstance that could have caused the condition.*

***Have any of your studies touched on hormonal links because it is a mostly female condition?***

*You would have to ask this question in a condition where the ratio of women to men is nine to one! Also people used to say that it is mostly post-menopausal women that develop takotsubo, but we have seen it across the whole age spectrum. I do not think that is necessarily anything related to menopause itself or post-menopause.*

***That information is still out there, though; they still do talk about it being a high percentage of post-menopausal women who suffer with takotsubo. Would you say that is maybe a little bit inaccurate now?***

*I would say it is a little speculative. Heart attacks are also more common in women after menopause, based on the concept that oestrogens are protective. However, all conditions become more common with age. We looked at the effect of HRT in our takotsubo registry but we did not see an association or a protective effect; however, the numbers of patients on HRT were very small.*

Expert opinions on takotsubo

*Is it quite common to be diagnosed with takotsubo even without experiencing chest pain or difficulty breathing?*

Yes, we see that. Some people just feel non-specifically unwell. It is often assumed that the patient is having a heart attack, so first-line health providers do an ECG and cardiac blood tests, and discover that something is going on with the heart.

*Is it possible for a takotsubo episode to cause a patient to have a heart attack?*

It is very difficult to answer this question. A heart attack is a stressor. So that can cause a takotsubo attack. The converse is something that we are looking to answer in the future, whether takotsubo unmasks a certain vulnerability for the cardiovascular system of a specific individual.

*So, in that case, if that were found to be a possibility, then we should be mindful of our lifestyle, as takotsubo patients?*

Possibly. It is very frustrating because there are still a lot of things that we do not know. We cannot give advice on the basis of no information and no knowledge.

*Have you seen a lot of people suffering with depression post takotsubo?*

It is one thing to have depressive illnesses; it is different to have a reactive depressive state because you feel that you want to get on with life, and this is stopping you from doing so. One could even call it impatience; frustration as well.

Initially it was thought takotsubo was associated with mental health conditions, but when we looked at large patient cohorts, we concluded there is no difference between the proportion *of patients who develop takotsubo and have a previously diagnosed mental health condition and the proportion of mental health conditions present in the general population.*

**Have you ever encountered a patient who had an event following a HIIT (high intensity interval training) session? Is this a form of exercise we should avoid?**

*We say to generally avoid stress but I would not say that HIIT training is stress; quite the opposite. It is good for health, it boosts the endorphins, it makes one happy. Can one avoid everything in life that could possibly lead to something like takotsubo? A lot of people we see have developed the condition at funerals. Does it mean one has to avoid funerals? You cannot, can you? Life goes on.*

# Chapter Fourteen

# Stories of takotsubo

In this chapter, a selection of takotsubo patients share their experiences. Below you will find a short glossary of terms used in these accounts:

**Troponin** is a protein that's found in the cells of the heart muscle. Normally, it stays inside the heart muscle's cells, but damage to those cells — such as the kind of damage from a heart attack — causes it to leak into the blood. The more damage there is to the heart, the greater the amount of troponin there will be in the blood. Troponin levels usually increase sharply within three to 12 hours after a heart attack and peak about 24 hours afterwards. They will also remain high for several days.

**Heart 'cath' or catheterisation, also known as an angiogram**
This is an invasive test used to detect heart problems. A long, thin tube (catheter) is inserted into your wrist or groin and guided up to your heart. A dye is then injected, allowing x-rays to capture pictures of the coronary arteries, thereby enabling closer inspection of any blockages or narrowings, and also to determine the condition of the heart valves and heart muscle.

**Echocardiogram**: This is an ultrasound image of the heart; it enables doctors to diagnose a range of heart problems.

**Atrial fibrillation**, also known as AF and Afib, is the most common heart rhythm disturbance. It develops in the heart's upper chambers, leading to irregular heartbeat. It can cause heart palpitations, dizziness, difficulty breathing, fatigue, chest pain and confusion. It is also known as **arrhythmia**, a common term for an abnormal heart rhythm.

**Bradycardia** is a slow heart rate. Adults usually have a heart rate between 60 and 100 beats per minute, but if you have bradycardia, your heart beats fewer than 60 times per minute.

**Tachycardia** is when the heart beats too fast, at a rate of more than 100 beats per minute, when at rest.

**Ejection fraction (EF)** refers to how well your heart pumps blood. It is a measure of the amount of blood pumped out of your heart's lower chambers (ventricles) each time they contract. To understand EF, it's helpful to have an idea, in simple terms, of how blood flows through the heart:

1. Blood enters the heart through the top right section (atrium).
2. Between heartbeats, there's a short pause. This is when blood flows through a valve down to the left ventricle.
3. Once the ventricle is full, the next heartbeat pumps (ejects) a portion of the blood out to the body.

EF in a healthy heart is approximately 50% to 70%. With each heartbeat, 50% to 70% of the blood in the left ventricle gets pumped out to the body. A low EF is typically 45% or less and can be evidence of heart failure or cardiomyopathy.

**Cardiomyopathy** is a general term meaning any disorder or disease that affects the heart muscle.

**Supraventricular tachycardia (SVT)** is an umbrella term for fast heart rhythms arising from the upper part of the heart, namely the left and right atria.

**NSTEMI heart attack:** A non-ST-elevation myocardial infarction (NSTEMI) is a type of heart attack. It causes a partial or incomplete blockage of one of the body's coronary arteries, reducing blood flow to the heart.

## Valerie's story

Valerie Anderson is aged 64 and lives in Tampa, Florida, USA. She is a wedding co-ordinator and owns an antiques business. This is her story:

> Before the takotsubo event, I worked seven days a week at my two businesses. I am a self-confessed workaholic. I ate healthily – I am basically a pescatarian – and had normal cholesterol and normal blood pressure. In September 2023, I went for a girls' weekend to Orlando with my two 32-year-old best friends. At our hotel was a huge water slide, and everything in my being said 'don't go down it'. But being 64 and stubborn, I went down. Halfway down I started to feel dizzy and disorientated.
>
> The waterslide landed in a whirlpool. In what seemed like an eternity, I was in the whirlpool; I couldn't breathe and couldn't figure out how to get out, although I am a good swimmer, and I was only in five feet of water.
>
> As I struggled underwater, I felt myself losing consciousness, and then suddenly I was being pulled out of the pool by a lifeguard. I felt very strange and, even though I knew something was terribly wrong – I had an inexplicable sense of doom – I decided to suck it up and go to dinner with my friends. I had no chest pain and no dizziness, but all of a sudden became very nauseous and

knew that I had to vomit. I was in the restroom for 15 minutes and was very sick. Crying, I asked my friends to call an Uber so we could go to the local Urgent Care so I could get hydrated. The Urgent Care did some blood work and told me I'd had a dry drowning.

I looked out of the window and saw an ambulance pull up. I said to the doctor, 'Wow, someone must be very sick'. He looked at me and said, 'Honey, you're having a heart attack'. I was taken to ICU, where an emotionless doctor came in my room and told my husband right in front of me that I probably wasn't going to make it. She said, 'Your troponin is 4000'. I looked at her and said, 'What the hell is that?'

The next morning they did a heart cath. The cardiologist at this small hospital in Davenport Florida was lovely. After the heart cath he told me I'd had a takotsubo event. 'Wow,' I said, 'That sounds exotic'. I was told my EF (ejection fraction) was 40. I said, 'Well that doesn't sound too bad'. I had no idea. The cardiologist told me, 'You'll be OK, but it will take some time. In fact I'm going to keep you one more day and let you go home tomorrow.' I was shocked – surely they were going to keep me longer than that!

For the first two weeks after the event, I felt distraught and terrified; almost immobilised. I was used to running two businesses and could usually keep up with all of my young staff. I felt such a loss of my former self, wondering if I would ever get back to that strong, energetic individual. I finally had to get on an anti-anxiety medication to keep myself sane. I should say at this point that I had never been on any medications in my 64 years.

After six weeks I went back to 12-hour days working as a wedding planner. Do I feel back to normal? Nope. But mentally

I know I'm living again! I take my meds and monitor my blood pressure. I'm tired and sometimes I get a little out of breath. But being around life and not wallowing in the fact that I had this event has helped me more than anything.

The gift that came out of all of this, for me, is that the sky looks a little bit bluer; the flowers look a little bit brighter; and I have a lot more patience and love for the people around me.

My advice for anyone going through this is to try to stay as positive as you can. Join a support group. Rest and truly take care of yourself first. And when you get depressed or anxious, get moving... walk, go shopping, visit a friend. Don't let the negative thoughts waste your precious time here.

## David's story

David B is aged 76, retired and lives in Accrington, Lancashire, in the UK. This is his story:

I have experienced and dealt with what might be seen as a fair number of traumas in my life, from being abandoned by my mother at the age of 13 months and subsequently spending most of the first five years of my life in a children's home; to my adult life when I experienced two divorces; my first wife's attempted suicide; and receiving psychiatric help for gambling and alcohol addiction.

I later got accepted to study Philosophy at the University of Leeds, graduating in 1995 with a 2(i) honours degree. After that, I spent my life in a perpetual round of drunkenness and debauchery until I met the woman who became (and is still some 22 years later) my third wife. Peggy Linda has, one might say, saved me from myself.

## What becomes of the broken-hearted

In 2011, I suffered a serious stroke, and since then, I have been inclined to get quite emotional and have developed a very sensitive nature and outlook.

In June 2024, I was having dental treatment which involved the removal of a broken molar under local anaesthetic. The procedure did not go according to plan and involved a lot of digging and drilling over a period of about 30 minutes. The surgeon used a considerable amount of force but eventually had to concede that she could not extract the tooth and root completely and stopped the procedure. By this time I was in a state of severe distress and I began to experience chest pains and tightness. A number of people from the dental practice were summoned, as was my wife who was waiting for me in the waiting room.

Someone in charge recognised that I was possibly having a cardiac event and paramedics were called and arrived quite quickly. After they carried out some tests I was rushed by ambulance to Royal Blackburn Teaching Hospital.

Over a period of four days I was closely monitored for blood pressure and heart beat. Blood samples were taken and I had an angiogram, after which takotsubo was diagnosed. I was discharged after four days and prescribed a number of medications including aspirin, statins, beta blockers and an angina spray.

After discharge I felt drained, very weak and depressed. I had no follow-up for TTS but I was re-admitted four weeks later with symptoms suggesting I had kidney and liver damage. Whilst it has not been confirmed that this episode was caused by the increased medication I was now taking (in addition to a fairly substantial amount of medication I was already on following the stroke), the consultant I was now under for my gastric problems authorised the cessation of most of the additional medication recently prescribed, and I began to get better.

I feel pretty much recovered from TTS, although I still tire easily and get breathless with even the slightest exertion.

My advice for anyone who has experienced this condition is to try not to worry, and to take it a day at a time.

## Claire's story

Claire Darlington was 60 when she had her first event, and 67 when she had her second. She is now aged 70 and lives in Warwickshire in the UK. She is a retired school teacher. This is her story:

It was a Thursday evening in May 2014 and I had been to my usual choir practice. After the practice ended, I stood in the car park talking to the pianist who is a friend of mine. We were discussing some unpleasantness there had been in the choir, starting a few months previously, with some rather unkind emails that had been sent. Finally, he said he was going home and I walked a few yards to the pub where I knew some of my choir friends had already gone.

As I walked to the pub I started to feel unwell. I felt a little bit shivery, even though it was a warm evening, and suddenly I started experiencing chest pain.

It wasn't too bad at first and it just felt like indigestion. After I reached the pub and sat down, the pain increased and I began to suspect it was not indigestion after all and, after refusing at first, I finally allowed my friend to ask the pub landlord to ring for an ambulance.

Paramedics arrived very quickly. My husband and son, having been alerted to the problem, arrived shortly afterwards. As the ambulance made its way to Coventry Hospital, the pain became so intense that the paramedic gave me intravenous morphine.

Immediately I arrived at the hospital I was met by a team of people. The consultant told me I was almost certainly having a heart attack. I was given aspirin and taken straight along to have an angiogram. The consultant then told me that I had not had a heart attack but something called 'takotsubo cardiomyopathy' and wrote it down on a piece of paper for me.

I think my first feeling was one of relief that it was not a heart attack but I felt confused by the diagnosis as I had never heard of it.

After I was discharged, I felt exhausted and had no energy at all. I felt relieved that I was still alive but worried that I would never feel my old self again. When I was told that it was usually caused by a very stressful event and/or extreme anxiety, I was puzzled. I have never suffered from depression, anxiety or stress.

University College Hospital prescribed bisoprolol (a beta-blocker) and clopidigrel (a blood-thinner), which they told me I should be on for a year, and referred me back to my local hospital. I had a follow-up appointment with the cardiologist there.

I felt that the Coventry doctors knew and understood the condition but the cardiologist at my local hospital appeared to know little about it and was not interested. A few months afterwards he told me I was fine (although all they had done that day was to test my blood pressure) and was dismissive when I told him I still had no energy. When I asked him when I could come off the medication, he told me I was now on it for life and recommended that I also start on statins. When I asked why, if I had, as he said, totally recovered, he just said vaguely that it was to protect my heart.

A year later I found a specialist in takotsubo in London and my GP, who was concerned by the lack of interest shown by the local cardiologist, immediately referred me to him. I had my first appointment with him in 2015 and I was so relieved to find someone who knew about the condition and was interested in me. For the first time I was asked to give a detailed account of what had happened before the event and he told me that I no longer needed to be on blood-thinners, beta-blockers or statins. I did feel rather better when I came off these.

Over the next few years I felt I was doing OK. My blood pressure was much higher than before my TTS so my medication was increased and I was reviewed by the TTS specialist every year.

In 2021 I had to have a minor procedure after developing mild vaginal bleeding. In the July I went into my local hospital to have a hysteroscopy under anaesthetic as it was suspected I had polyps. The doctor and anaesthetist were aware of my past TTS. I wasn't worried. In 2015 I had had a partial knee replacement and in 2017, as the first one had failed, I had had a full replacement in revision surgery. Neither time had I had any heart issues. However, when I woke up in the recovery room after the hysteroscopy, I started to have a dragging feeling down my left arm. Within a couple of minutes a cardiac nurse was by my side giving me an ECG. I was then told I was having a heart attack and was being blue-lighted to Coventry. In Resusc, I was given another ECG and blood tests which confirmed that my troponin level was very high. However, I did not feel too unwell and certainly did not have the extreme pain I had experienced the first time. An angiogram performed later confirmed I had had a second takotsubo episode.

I was stunned to have another TTS. I just thought I never would. I was getting on with my life and enjoying retirement. Despite the fact that this TTS was so much milder than the first, it has actually left me with more issues. I am, however, determined not to let having had two takotsubos define my life.

As for advice to others going through this, finding a cardiologist who understands the condition certainly helps. I found mine to be very reassuring. I do believe that thinking positively is important. If you let TTS define who you are, you never move on. I try not to get too hung up on my blood pressure as I am sure worrying about it is only likely to make it worse. Meeting up with friends and enjoying life is really important. I have tried not to let TTS affect my outlook on life, but, inevitably, it does to some extent. However, I feel lucky to be alive and am determined to enjoy whatever time I have left.

## Marian's story

Marian is aged 75 and lives in Cornwall in the UK. She is a retired local government officer. This is her story:

I had COVID in January 2020, which left me with chronic IBS. I isolated myself during lockdown and continued to do so after lockdown was lifted due to my fear of getting COVID again. During those three years I had problems with a neighbour who was abusive, trespassing and damaging my property. Also during that time my husband had an affair. On the day of my event, in May 2023, I had been sitting in the sun in my garden all day as I felt unwell. When I got up to go into my house at 6:00 pm I saw that the neighbour had leant over my garden fence and cut the top off my tree. My thoughts were that the trouble was escalating again. Immediately I felt breathless, choking, unable to breathe and had pain in my chest going over my shoulder, into my back, down my arm and up into my jaw. I felt I might pass out.

I thought I was having an asthma attack, so took my ventolin inhaler. I didn't feel any better, my heart was racing, so thought it could be a panic attack. I meditated for a short time. Still not feeling better, I took my blood pressure which was 200+/113. I phoned NHS 111 and asked for advice. I was informed an emergency ambulance would be sent to me. When the paramedics arrived, I was treated with a GTN (glyceryl trinitrate – see page 162) spray and felt a little better; I could breathe more easily. I was taken to A&E and admitted to a medical assessment unit.

I had an echocardiogram on the second day of my hospital stay, and was told that my heart had been damaged. I was diagnosed with heart failure, following what the consultant thought was a heart attack. On day 10, I had an angiogram and was told that I had 'takotsubo cardiomyopathy', or 'broken heart syndrome'. I had never heard of it.

I didn't believe what had happened to me at first. I was sure there was nothing seriously wrong. After a few days in hospital, I accepted my diagnosis, but I was shocked, frightened and tearful.

I was discharged after 11 days, but I felt sad, frightened and totally alone with my fears. I was exhausted and upset that I couldn't carry out my normal household chores and gardening.

At first my husband thought I was 'cured' and back to normal. He realised after Googling 'takotsubo' that he was wrong and has since been fully supportive. He tells me to rest and has taken over some of the household chores and gardening. I don't think he understood initially what had happened to me, as I didn't understand either. My friends were shocked as I have always been active, but they were very supportive and caring.

I was discharged from hospital on five different medications and informed that I would have a further echocardiogram in three months. I contacted my GP to discuss my condition and he reassured me that the cardiologist expected my heart to make a full recovery. The week following my discharge I received a phone call from a Cardiac Nurse. She reassured me that my heart could recover fully but advised that some people's hearts do not. She monitored my blood pressure and weight daily (which I took at home and relayed to her) for two weeks. I was able to phone her when I was worried, and this was very helpful. She referred me to a Counsellor because I was tearful and frightened.

I am not back to full strength yet. It takes me much longer to carry out my daily tasks, but mentally I am much better; I am having counselling, and I am much more positive about life.

I have followed a vegan diet for 40 years, but on the advice of the dietitian when I was in hospital, I have added more protein and calcium products to my diet. (I had not been eating much prior to my event since I had little appetite.)

I take things slowly and don't push myself anymore. I can't do all the things I used to do (i.e., gardening, DIY, spring cleaning). I have given up perfectionism. I try not to get stressed by meditating and not taking part in any confrontation. I don't socialise like I used to. I meet my friends through zoom.

My advice for others going through this is to rest as much as possible after diagnosis, take things slowly and don't be impatient about recovery. It takes time to get well again. Eat well, sleep, join a takotsubo group and learn from others who have the condition. Seek counselling if frightened. Meditate if possible; accept support and help from your friends and family. You will get better.

## Alex's story

Alex Scott is aged 66 and lives in Quebec, Canada. She is a dual Canadian-American. This is her story:

In 2008, I founded an environmental organisation in St Mary's, Georgia, USA, and worked as its director until 2021 when I moved to Quebec. It was a challenging job, complete with high-profile battles galore and my very own death-threat-spewing stalker. During those years, I continued as a freelance writer and occasionally served as a personal trainer at the local gym. I still serve on the Executive Committee of the Okefenokee Protection Alliance (representing over five million members). In 2018, I had (what was deemed at the time) a mild heart attack - with no discernible cause.

In the summer of 2023, at the time of the takotsubo event, I was recently retired... for the most part.

We were staying at our cabin in the middle of Nantahala National Forest in North Carolina (elevation: 5000 ft). I was relaxed, happy and healthy. I'm a life-long vegetarian, 5'2" tall, 107 lb, and a fitness buff who loves hiking and gyms. In short, there was no 'trigger' that I can think of.

## What becomes of the broken-hearted

We'd walked down to a lookout and were hiking back up a long and fairly steep incline. I began to feel my heart racing, shortness of breath, and nausea. So, me being me, I paused for a moment and then continued on. Then paused then continued. Then paused. The darkness began to close in around the edges of my vision and there was a sharp pain between my shoulder blades. I informed my partner and best friend that I needed to 'sit for a bit', plomped myself down in the dirt, turned onto my side, and neatly vomited in the road.

For the next 30 minutes, I passed in and out of consciousness. My heart rate dropped down into the low 30s and my companions summoned an ambulance. Due to the remote location, it took another 30 minutes for help to arrive. I felt quite relaxed as I drifted in the dirt, in the arms of my partner and friend, and waited to die. For some reason, I was rather serene about it all: perhaps the trials of the 'heart attack', getting through the COVID times, a divorce, an international move, and a lifetime of accumulated emotional trauma had rendered me a tad fatigued.

Finally, I was loaded into an ambulance and taken to an airfield where a Medivac helicopter gobbled me up and whisked me off to Mission Hospital in Asheville, North Carolina.

My troponin level was high (11) and my ejection fraction (EF) was low (35). I had an echocardiogram, after which the cardiologist informed me that I had something called 'takotsubo syndrome' and carefully explained what had happened. I'd never heard of such a thing.

What they couldn't tell me was why it had happened. Or how to avoid having it happen again. Or what it meant for my life. Or how to go on while knowing that my heart could blow up while I was folding towels or playing with my grandson or crying over a sad film or laughing at my dog's antics or falling in love or grieving the loss of a friend or greeting spring or breathing.

Five days later, I was discharged... without any instructions other than that I should contact my own cardiologist. So, I simply returned to my usual habits. Three days after discharge, I flew home across the country, walked my dog each day for about five miles, and carried on as if nothing had happened.

About a month after the event, I had an echocardiogram which revealed that my heart was 'back to normal' and my EF was 65. The cardiologist's only instructions were, 'Go out and live your best life'.

My friends and family are, understandably, shaken and worried. I'm sure that I frustrate and confuse them by my insistence that I simply go on as if nothing has changed – but what has, really, other than that I take a couple more pills each day and can't really count on a future?

Yes, I get scared in the deep of night sometimes if I wake up and my heart feels heavy or I'm running up the stairs and I experience a twinge in my upper back. 'Is this it? Is it happening again?'

And I'm angry. If I'm given logical sequences to work with (A led to B which led to C which resulted in D), I can deal with almost anything. But this feels as if the hand of a capricious god reached down from the skies – or up from the bowels of the earth – plunged into my chest, and reshaped my heart.

My job now is to live as fully and as well as I can. More fully and better than ever before. Because I'll be damned if I'm going to creep through my days and nights in fear of being turned back into an octopus pot.

## Elinor's story

Elinor Gonzales is aged 29 and lives near Manila, Philippines. She is a nurse and business owner. This is her story:

When my takotsubo (TTS) happened, I was a healthy young woman of 29, although at 25 I had undergone surgery to donate my kidney to my dad.

The TTS happened in 2020, during COVID year. I was driving on my way home with my mom to pick up my dad to take him to the barber's shop. A few minutes before reaching our home, I suddenly felt my throat tighten a bit, and I had to cough a few times. Then I felt like I couldn't breathe. I slowed down and, as I reached the parking lot, a stabbing pain in my chest began. I thought I was having a heart attack. Back then, during the pandemic, a lot of young men and women suddenly died because of stroke, heart attack or cancer. I thought, 'Am I going to be one of them?'

Then the pain radiated to my shoulder down to my left arm and my fingers. I tried meditating, thinking to myself, 'Maybe I am just having a panic attack. I just need to be calm.' I was counting slowly, deep breathing and calming my mind. Nothing worked. It all happened in a few minutes. I asked my parents to take me to the ER. During the ride, my heart kept pounding, it was really painful, I couldn't breathe, I thought my chest was going to explode. I was so afraid that my heart wouldn't handle the fast heartbeat and would just stop beating.

As we reached the hospital, my aunt, who is a doctor in that hospital, was waiting for us at the entrance of the ER. They took me in, gave me oxygen, and did an ECG. My heart rate was at 189 bpm, more than three times the normal rate. I was lying down on the bed, and I could feel my heart pounding, so loud that it felt like the bed was moving, like an earthquake.

Being my optimistic, strong self, I acted like nothing happened. I even walked to the restroom to pee as if I was OK. I joked around saying, 'I guess God doesn't want me in Heaven yet', but deep inside I was petrified. They asked me if I wanted to be admitted. I refused, scared I might get COVID in the hospital. So I just had a 2D echo [echocardiogram] that day and left for home.

In the third or fourth month after my attack, around March 2021, I was ordered to take another 2D echo test. With my results, I went to the cardiologist and to my surprise, everything was back to normal. She proceeded to ask if there was a stressful event that had happened to me. With my mom being in the room, I couldn't answer because, truthfully, there was, but I had been doing my best not to show it. She told me that it was 'takotsubo' or 'broken heart syndrome'; I couldn't believe what I heard. It's just something that we had studied at nursing school: emotional pain turning into physical pain.

As I went home, I thought about what had happened to me. I had detached from the stress I was experiencing; I tried not to show it; but as I thought about the series of events leading up to December 8th, I understood why it happened.

Back in 2019, two years after our successful kidney transplant, my dad had been diagnosed with liver cancer. It was a huge blow for us. He underwent surgery and we thought everything was fine. But a few months before my attack, his check-ups had been showing signs of recurrence. Although it wasn't confirmed yet, I guess it was always in the back of my mind. Also, four months before my attack, August 2020, my boyfriend of six years and I broke up.

I refused to share any thoughts or emotions with my family, thinking that it would hurt them to see me in pain. We were in lockdown, too, because of COVID, so I couldn't go out and see friends to lighten up. I would cry alone in my room or in the shower, and would turn my face away whenever they were around. My mum always thought that I was so strong. A week after our break-up, a dear friend of mine suddenly died of a heart attack. I was crushed. I lost too much in a span of a week. I didn't know what to do but to just work and work and to keep my mind busy; pushing all my emotions aside. Then in November 2020, I was diagnosed with an ovarian cyst, which was a big blow to me as well because I thought I would have difficulty bearing children someday. Then a couple of days before my attack, my dad's cancer was confirmed to have a recurrence. All of these events happened, and through it all I never allowed my family to see me cry. I guess my defence mechanism has always been detachment. I needed to do it, I had to, somebody needs to be strong and move and make important decisions logically without emotions. But I guess my body was telling me otherwise.

The TTS has affected my life, because I know now how it can happen. I finally understand the importance of releasing emotions and stress. I have been more at peace with how I take sudden news. I am grateful for the events that happened to me, as since then I have learned the power of faith and self-awareness. I hope this brings light to everyone who has gone through takotsubo and its triggering event. You are not alone. Take care of yourself, listen to your body more and know that you will get through it stronger and wiser.

## Lori's story

Lori Fieger is aged 53 and lives in Anaheim, California, in the USA. She works as a para-educator. This is her story:

I was 50 and extremely healthy when this happened to me. Over Christmas, I damaged my right knee and was in pain from that, so in January I saw an orthopaedist who gave me a cortisone shot in my knee. I spent the next day resting because I was exhausted and in pain. At 5:00 pm that day I went from feeling not great to feeling awful. All at once my bra was too tight, so I tried to remove it. The movement made me feel dizzy and nauseous, so I attempted to get to the bathroom before I threw up. But my eyesight was blurry and wiggly so I sat back down. It felt like someone was sitting on the top of my chest. It also felt like when Bugs Bunny saw a girl bunny – I could feel my heart beating outside my chest like it was trying to fly away, so I was holding it in my chest with my hands. I had no energy and my skin turned grey. I was clammy all over. I also felt muddled and confused.

I couldn't think straight, was incredibly weak, and didn't have my phone beside me, so I was stuck in my chair until my husband came home from work and noticed me. He saw I was the same colour as my chair (grey) and began asking me questions. We have a blood pressure cuff at home; he got that on me quickly. 182/128 mm Hg was the highest reading at home. Once he saw my BP was not coming down, he called the paramedics.

I was all the wrong things: a white 50-year-old female presenting with a heart attack who did NOT have COVID... it took a few phone calls (15-20 minutes) before they found a hospital that would take me.

Upon admittance to the hospital I spent the first 14+ hours in the makeshift parking garage 'wing' (think of a MASH episode – it was COVID) receiving fantastic care.

I was finally taken into hospital to go into the cath lab for my angiogram where they found zero blockages. I also had chest x-rays. My troponin levels were elevated; they kept checking that all weekend, plus lots of other bloodwork. From that point on I was in the hospital itself until my release two days later.

At the end of my stay a doctor came in and told me I had not had a heart attack; I had had a 'takotsubo event'. He didn't know that much about it – it was not his speciality.

I'd never heard of it before and spent some time looking it up and being confused by all the seemingly different info out there.

I was released with a handful of blood pressure and other meds; until that point I'd not been on any prescription medication.

I am the only takotsubo patient my cardiologist has. He's kind enough, but his knowledge is limited and outdated. I have tried to share what I've learned with him, but it doesn't seem to hold weight because I am not a doctor.

I was shocked by having a 'heart attack' because I'd always been very healthy, but I was, and remain, simply happy to be alive.

My energy level will probably never return to where it was before, but I am fine with 70-80% of my former energy.

I am back at work part time and occasionally sub. Most days I have energy to spare, but if I don't, I've learned how to listen to my body better than I ever had before. And I care for myself in real time. I am thankful for that knowledge.

I eat more healthily than before – my own blend of Mediterranean and vegetarian, although I do eat chicken, turkey and fish. Gone are breads, pastas and sweets, except on special occasions.

My advice for other TTS survivors is to allow yourself to recover and be gracious to your body as you do so; don't worry about how long recovery takes – yours is unique to you; learn to hear what your body is telling you; be real with yourself and others about myriad feelings you experience; and embrace your 'new normal' with a joyful heart every day; and continue living each day to the fullest. Take the second (or third or fourth) chance you've been given and live life with gusto. I no longer take any day for granted. I doubt I ever will again.

## Anita's story

Anita Johnsson is aged 55 and lives in Östersund, in the north of Sweden. She works in elderly homecare and is a full-time student. This is her story:

Before the takotsubo event I was in good health. In July of 2023 my mother got ill and passed away within three weeks. At the same time my father had surgery for cancer; the weekend after that, his sister died, and a month later his other sister died too. So we had three funerals within two months.

I had been stressed about all of this during late summer, and occasionally I felt anxiety, with slight pressure on the chest, and the feeling of not getting enough air.

The takotsubo event occurred during a skiing tour in the woods with my sister and our dogs in November of 2023. I suddenly felt very tired, and at first I didn't understand what was going on, so I continued skiing until we got back to the car. This was really stupid.

After resting for a while, it was suddenly like someone pulled the plug. I had foggy sight, was extremely weak, had chest pain that led down into my left arm and my throat, and the feeling of not getting enough air.

My sister drove to the local health centre, were they took blood and gave me an ECG. My blood was high in troponin, and my blood pressure was 107/68 mm Hg, so fairly low. The ECG was normal. From there I went by ambulance to the hospital, where they did a coronary x-ray.

The coronary x-ray showed that my arteries looked fine, but they diagnosed takotsubo due to the shape of my heart. I was sad, and scared, and ashamed. I thought I had brought this on myself. I had heard of broken heart syndrome, but really didn't know anything about it.

After being discharged from hospital, I was physically weak. I got exhausted just walking from the car to the house. Mentally I had a wake-up call. I understood that I had to reconsider life, and value the things that are important if I want to be in it for a long time. I also felt quite fragile and insecure, and did not want to be alone.

I had no follow-up care at first. I have called the hospital to make contact with the physiotherapist connected to cardio.

I am still weak physically, but it is getting better day by day. Mentally I feel worried, sad and lonely.

My advice to anyone who has been through this is to seek

someone to talk to, a therapist, and see that you get help both mentally and physically. I am rethinking and re-evaluating my life, and that's quite some work.

## Barbara's story

Barbara* is aged 73 and lives in Flanders, Belgium. This is her story:

As a child I loved roller skating, climbing trees, playing football on the street, swimming and cycling. As a teenager I enjoyed horse riding and judo, reaching European level, and going on to practise for 30 years. I started jogging at 23 until I was 55, when I had to stop due to knee problems. From then on it was cycling on the home trainer on a regular basis. At 60, I started Pilates twice a week and added fitness training later on. As you can tell, I love to move!

I was lucky to be in good health, with normal BMI, normal cholesterol values, no high blood pressure and no diabetes. I never smoked, and drank alcohol very moderately. As my partner had had heart bypass surgery, I had also followed a 'low fat' and 'low sugar' diet for the past 12 years. In fact, my physical condition, when I was tested aged 61, was considered to be 'excellent' for my age. My average daily steps totalled around 12,000.

And then COVID hit. From March 2020, almost all my fitness activities were curtailed and my daily steps reduced to around 7000-8000.

*Barbara's name has been changed.

## What becomes of the broken-hearted

It was Friday 19th of November 2021 when my life changed. On that day I had a personal training session. I completed a circuit training, but found that the HIIT (high intensity interval training) on the exercise bike felt very strenuous and made me out of breath. As I finished the second round, I felt exhausted. I started to walk home and about five minutes later I started to feel a sharp, though bearable, pain behind the sternum. It lasted five or six hours and I didn't think too much about it. I didn't sleep very well, however, and the following days there was still a pain, if milder. I still wasn't too concerned and continued my business, even driving 150 km for a meeting on the Monday. I did not mention my symptoms to my partner because he had some health problems of his own and is prone to worrying.

However, my sleep was still not good, and also I noticed that my resting heart rate was rising day after day. I have had a fitness tracking device since 2015, so I knew quite well what my normal values were. Then I got worried and was wondering about a 'silent heart attack'. It was still 'COVID time' and not as easy to obtain a consultation with a GP as it usually was in Belgium. Furthermore, I wanted an ECG done, and was not sure if a GP could do this. So I told my partner: 'Don't worry, but I am just going to the Emergency Department of our local clinic because I want to have something checked out.' And then I drove to the ER.

Arriving in the ER on the fifth day after the onset of the symptoms, I was immediately seen to as I was 'Tachy' (heart rate >100 bpm). A nurse took some blood and I had an ECG. Around 15 minutes later the ER doctor came and told me: 'I don't see anything wrong on your ECG, but we'll wait to see what the blood analysis shows.' So I phoned my partner and told him to be patient for a while and not to be concerned as the ECG seemed OK.

About an hour later, another doctor came along and said: 'You do have some slightly raised "heart enzymes" in your blood, so we will run some tests.' (In fact, my troponin values were raised but I did not know that at the time.) A trainee cardiologist came in and started questioning me: What had happened? Did I have health problems? Did someone in my family have heart problems? I said no, and explained that I was worried about the possibility of a silent heart attack although I didn't seem to tick any of the boxes... He agreed, and informed me that to be sure I would need an angiogram in a catheter lab. Then he looked rather curiously at me and said, 'You seem to be a very reasonable woman, not nervous or anxious, so did you have chemo in the past?' I had no idea what this conversation meant.

Two hours later an echo was done; and it was then explained to me: 'See here; you can see an abnormal wall movement; this is very clear. You have "broken heart syndrome". This is a condition that does not last and in a few weeks you'll be OK again.'

I was so shocked by my diagnosis. I felt an intense grief for my sudden lost health, and I went through all stages from denial to anger to acceptance (over time). It gradually became clear to me that what had happened to me was not something like a sprained ankle, but something more serious with possible lasting complications. The thought that the causes and the therapy were not well known and that recurrence, although not likely, was not to be excluded was not helpful either.

I immediately made an appointment to write my last will and testament as I am childless and unmarried. After that was finished, a strange feeling of calm and peace came over me. I reflected on my life and felt content. This, however, did not last long. Life was pulling on my sleeve and wanted to be lived. Day to day activities were not so much of a problem, but I had some unexplained bouts of fatigue that would spring up and make me lie down for an hour or so, and I had to ask my partner to be very gentle with me as the slightest remark from him would give me some pain behind the sternum.

Sports being my passion, I was worried about my risks, especially as I presumed the trigger in my case was exercise. It took a while before I went to my first Pilates session. The idea of doing a cycling test on my next medical follow-up after four months frankly terrified me. There was a real loss of confidence I had never experienced before. At the same time I felt sorry because going to the point of exhaustion in sports had always given me such a 'good feeling'. Endomorphs, I guess.

Talking and explaining to friends and relatives was really helpful. Most of them had never heard of the condition and listened with interest. Being a scientist, I plunged into the medical literature; I felt comforted by not being alone with my questions and fears.

After 10 months I had my third follow-up. In the discussion with the cardiologist, I mentioned that I still had bouts of fatigue and sometimes a burning sensation behind the sternum. In the end he told me: 'By now, you probably know more about the condition than I do.' I thought this was very honest of him but not very reassuring!

I am grateful to live in a country where the healthcare is very well organised and affordable. My mentality changed and I became 'milder' towards myself and people in general. I accepted that I could not perform as well as I had done in the past and I tried to adapt my lifestyle accordingly, without feeling guilty.

My advice to anyone who suspects TTS: Do not hesitate to go to an ER department and insist on a proper diagnosis. Secondly I would say, gather as much information as possible from reliable sources about the syndrome, don't panic but observe how you feel calmly; talk about it with family and friends and be aware that it may take a long time to recover – but don't give up.

## Alexandra's story

Alexandra is aged 65 and lives in Northern Illinois in the USA. She is a retired cyber security analyst. This is her story:

At the end of January 2021, one evening I was relaxing on the couch, watching television. I leaned forward to get the remote to change the channel. After changing the channel, I leaned back, with my feet raised on a foot rest. I felt a strong shock, or vibration, internally throughout my entire body. No pain. Just the shock/vibration sensation. It was something that I had never felt before. I happened to be wearing an Apple Smartwatch. I checked my heart rate. It was rapidly rising.

There is a history of heart disease and blood clots in my family, and since I take high blood pressure medicine, I got up to get my blood pressure machine. When I took my blood pressure, it was at a critical level: 220/110 mm Hg. I knew something was wrong, so I called an ambulance. The paramedics took an ECG but nothing appeared abnormal. Only a high heart rate and high blood pressure. So I had my husband drive me to the hospital.

When I arrived at the ER, I waited in line, signed in, and waited to be called for about 15 minutes. After getting called into a room and explaining what had happened, my blood was tested. A little while later, I was rushed into another room because the blood tests indicated that I might be having a heart attack and/or a blood clot. I had very high troponin and d-dimer levels. (An elevated D-dimer level suggests an increased risk of a blood clot.) Then a battery of additional tests began that kept me up until 3:00 am.

I was extremely confused. I felt relatively fine. The doctors kept asking me – constantly – about chest pains. I didn't have any. Just a slight pressure near my upper left shoulder. So they put a nitro patch on that spot. That really didn't do anything for me. I didn't match their profile for a 'heart attack'. I was diagnosed with 'takotsubo' following an angiogram. I had never heard of it.

I was in the hospital for three days. They ran every test they could think of trying to figure out how this had happened. They came up empty-handed.

After discharge, I was tired, but that initially was it. Side-effects from some of the medications kicked in, but changes to my prescriptions cleared those up. I was confused because there wasn't an explanation for the takotsubo.

The doctors did not understand takotsubo at all. The male doctors stated, 'It's not serious'; 'You'll be fine'; 'You need to learn to relax'. (Seriously? I was relaxing on my couch when it happened!) I would call the cardiologist office (for three months afterwards, I had acute critical high blood pressure attacks with tachycardia), but I didn't feel anyone was really listening to me, or could answer my questions. I switched cardiologists, but my current cardio, who is a very good heart doctor, classifies me as a heart failure patient. All my echocardiograms after the TTS event have been normal, I have no symptoms of heart failure, yet I am permanently labeled a 'heart failure patient' on my medical records and treated as such. I think because so little is known about takotsubo, which affects treatment methods, cardiologists can only treat what they know, putting those of us who have suffered a TTS event in a bucket with heart attack patients where we don't belong.

My advice for anyone going through this is to be your own advocate. Join a support group if one exists. The doctors are busy so sometimes they aren't the best listeners and might not keep up on the latest research. The best experts about an illness or disease are usually those who have actually experienced the illness themselves.

## Lee Ann's story

Lee Ann Clemons is aged 64 and lives in South Texas, USA. She is a retired Director of Children's Ministries at First United Methodist Church in McAllen, Texas. This is her story:

It was October 2022. I was visiting with close family friends, comforting them following the death of one of the young adults in their family. As I was hugging the grandmother, whom I have always had a strong connection to, I experienced a feeling of discomfort rise in my chest.

I went straight over to my general doctor's office. After checking my blood pressure, he suggested I make another appointment with the cardiologist. I went home, but the discomfort stayed with me, and moved to my back. After three hours, I called my general doctor, and he told me to go to the Emergency Room. I was seen immediately upon arriving. An ECG was done, which was normal. Blood tests were done and very high troponin levels were identified. Chest x-ray was done which indicated emphysema, but turned out not to be an issue. The ER staff were suggesting it was a heart attack, but said more tests would be done to confirm that. I was eventually admitted and placed in a room. Blood tests continued and my troponin levels started to go down. I was given fluids and medications but was not sure what they were.

I was visited by a cardiologist on the morning following and, after hearing my story, he suggested that I might have experienced takotsubo cardiomyopathy or 'broken heart syndrome'. After that, an echocardiogram confirmed the low ejection fraction (24) and the swollen left ventricle. This was followed by an angiogram which showed no artery blockages... further confirmation of takotsubo.

I was very surprised having not heard of this before and having felt like I was in good health. I also felt relief that it was not a heart attack and no surgery would have to be performed. Also, my doctor gave me hope that this normally does not occur again and the heart goes back to normal in a short amount of time.

I had heard of broken heart syndrome, but only as it related to people having 'heart attacks' following extreme emotional stress. I had never heard of the terms takotsubo or takotsubo cardiomyopathy.

Following discharge from hospital, I felt very tired, had continued discomfort in my chest and heart palpitations. I had an extremely dry mouth, wobbly legs/feet, maybe from the medications or as a result of the takotsubo. Mentally I was quite fearful.

Several pills were prescribed as I left the hospital. As I went to my follow-up appointment with the cardiologist who had diagnosed the TTS in the hospital, he took me off of most of the medications and even implied that I really did not need to take anything. He ended up having me stay on a beta-blocker and aspirin. He said that I could go back to normal activity. He did not give me any information about what to expect in the months ahead. In addition, his office was very difficult to get in touch with, and I became quite anxious and unable to get answers to questions I had.

It is one year and one month since my event and I am finally feeling almost like I did before the TTS happened. I do still feel a little bit of discomfort in my chest from time to time, but I am so much better, still on a low dosage of beta-blocker but so much better. I am walking 30 minutes a day, when I could barely walk for 5 minutes after the TTS. I have gained back the 15lb that I lost following the event.

Mentally, I am so much better as well. After the TTS I was very fearful about whether it would happen again; if I would ever feel better. I saw a psychiatrist three times, started taking a low dose (2.5) of escitalopram, and had about six to eight sessions with a counsellor. I had heard about eye movement desensitisation and reprocessing therapy, EMDR, as a tool to help in coping with trauma and how it had been useful for people recovering from takotsubo. I specifically sought out a counsellor with certification in EMDR. Those sessions were extremely helpful in coping with the mental/emotional/psychological aspects of the TTS.

I also incorporated restorative yoga practice, breathing and meditative exercises and prayer into my recovery. All of these things worked together to help me mentally and physically. Considering the direct correlation between the brain, heart and stomach makes the use of these tools important and, in my case, necessary to my full recovery. In addition, the takotsubo support group on Facebook was and continues to be very helpful and gives me hope and the assurance that I am not alone.

I am more mindful now of my body and mind. I decided to retire from my busy job working with children in my church. I now am back to volunteering and can pick and choose what I want to be involved in. I make sure that my days are meaningful and spent with the people and activities that bring me joy and peace.

If you are going through this, my advice is to reach out to others who have experienced takotsubo. Find a doctor who has knowledge and experience of patients with it and one who is a good communicator and listener. Do your best to educate your family and friends about it, so they will understand what is going on with you. Seek out as many tools as you can find to help with the psychological aspects of your recovery. Know that every person's recovery will be different... be patient with yourself, listen to your heart, and rest!

## Carol's story

Carol O'Neill is aged 57 and lives in Dundee, Scotland. She is a team leader with a local charity. This is her story:

It was November 2021, and I was 55. I had been asked to go into the office to cover a peer support session. I was responsible for unlocking the building, deactivating the alarm system, setting up the room we were to be using and then holding the session.

I arrived at the building, deactivated the alarm in the area I was to be working in and began to set up the room. I then went to unlock the main door; as I tried to turn the key in the lock, I got a shooting pain from my wrist up to my shoulder. I gave my arm a shake and the pain disappeared. I then tried again to unlock the door and the pain shot up my arm again. The pain was such that it brought tears to my eyes and took my breath away. At that point I gave up trying to unlock the door and then walked a few steps to the reception desk to put the keys down as my wrist and arm were extremely sore. I consider that I have quite a high pain threshold but suddenly I experienced a severe pain in my throat; sweating; nausea; pain between the shoulder blades; a heavy feeling in my upper arms; I felt weak and needed to sit down; I also felt short of breath.

I video-called my manager to let her know what was happening – my intention was to go home and sleep it off. Once I was on the call, I could see my face was grey and beaded with sweat. When I saw this, I thought I was having a heart attack. I asked my manager to call an ambulance.

After being admitted to hospital and undergoing copious testing, an angiogram confirmed a diagnosis of takotsubo cardiomyopathy.

I was initially relieved by the diagnosis, as coronary heart disease is in our family history (my dad had his first cardiac arrest in his mid/late 30s; had a quadruple by-pass when he was 50; and died of a cardiac arrest when he was 63) and after my angiogram I was advised I only had slight furring of the arteries, so to me that was good news. I was also told there would be no lasting effects and that I would recover fully and was unlikely to have another takotsubo event.

I hadn't heard of takotsubo, but back in the 70s, I had had a friend at school whose grandad had died first and then her gran had died a couple of weeks later of a 'broken heart'. This was of course before anything was really known about TTS.

I do not feel that TTS was understood fully at the hospital. After my MRI, at a consultation afterwards, the cardiologist told me I'd had 'an old fashioned heart attack'. He also advised that I would be back to normal in four weeks. (It's now more than two years since the event and I'm still not back to normal.) I can only assume that his knowledge was poor and that it was easier for him to tell me I'd had a heart attack and discharge me from his care than to have to face me in the future. However, my GP has been amazing.

I still feel extremely fatigued – I need at least 10 hours of sleep each night, and ideally an afternoon nap for an hour or two also. I still have shortness of breath, though it has improved, but I still can't walk and talk at the same time; and I have to walk very slowly.

I can't do, physically, what I was able to do prior to the takotsubo event but at least I'm alive and I have learned to ask for help from others.

Mentally I'm not too bad, although I do get a bit frightened if I get similar symptoms; I wonder if all the medications are necessary but I'm too scared to stop any of them in case that's tempting fate; I get frustrated that my life has changed so much and I have to rely on others.

On a positive note, I no longer feel guilty saying no to people – my health has to come first. My new grandson certainly gives me the determination to keep going.

## Julia's story

Julia is 68 years old and lives in the Southeastern USA. This is her story:

My first encounter with heart problems was in late 2021, a little over a year before my takotsubo cardiomyopathy (TTS) event. Prior to that, I was on no medications and was relatively healthy.

I was getting ready to walk in the morning, but I felt vaguely ill and tense. I took my pulse, and it was 140 bpm and irregular. I then took my blood pressure (BP) and it was 185/110 mm Hg. (Normal is between 90/60 and 120/80.) I checked my blood pressure periodically, and it had never been high. I went to the ER where they did an ECG right away, which showed supraventricular tachycardia (SVT) (oddly, no one else was in the waiting room!), and they took me immediately back to a monitored bed. A cardiologist did come to see me and did a complete history and physical in the ER. The arrythmia was successfully converted and my heart rate and BP came down with intravenous (IV) diltiazem and IV metoprolol. I stayed in the hospital overnight where I had a chest x-ray, an echocardiogram and a cardiac stress test as well as another thyroid function test; they were all normal. I was put on oral forms of the IV medications and sent home the next day with follow up with the cardiology nurse practitioner that week.

Unfortunately, when I had my takotsubo event in early 2023, the ER was packed. I had gone to church that evening where I had Mexican food with a brownie and ice cream. I came home to watch my favourite TV shows, but being a little tired, I accidentally took a second dose of my diltiazem instead of my nightly metoprolol. I had done this once previously with no problems after checking with the cardiologist on call.

About two hours later, I felt very tense and took my blood pressure which was 198/135 mm Hg and my heart rate was 150 bpm and regular. I called a neighbour to take me to the ER. After 15 minutes, I was called to have an ECG and blood work. After about an hour in the waiting room, I developed chest pain, shortness of breath and left-sided numbness on my face. I went and told the triage nurse about these symptoms, and she told me to sit back down in the waiting room. I demanded that they take my vital signs again, which were still abnormal.

I got in touch with the on-call cardiologist by phone and went back to the triage nurse who was talking to him. At this point, I was past the 'golden hour' for intervention for a coronary blockage and was quite concerned as my chest pain and shortness of breath worsened. I was also concerned about having a stroke with my high blood pressure. I waited five more hours in the waiting room with chest pain and shortness of breath and two more hours in a monitored bed in the ER without being seen by a physician or having a chest x-ray. I was almost the last person to be taken into the ER from the waiting room!

When my second troponin came back at 300 and a re-check came back at over 1000, everyone sprang into action. I had come in at about 8:00 pm and it was now almost 7:00 am the next day. I was immediately prepped for cardiac catheterisation with defibrillating pads, three IVs, including a nitroglycerin drip. I had to ask for oxygen as I was still short of breath. The hospitalist who was going to admit me after my catheterisation came to see me and introduced himself, but I never saw the ER physician after being there for almost two hours.

I was blissfully sedated with fentanyl for my catheterisation and was woken up 10 minutes later by the cardiologist, who told me that my coronary arteries were clear, but that I had classic takotsubo cardiomyopathy with an ejection fraction (EF) of 20-25% (confirmed later by echocardiogram).

Since I had been an ICU nurse many years before, I knew that an EF that low was serious. I spent five days on the cardiac floor of the hospital where I developed chest pain and mild respiratory distress.

Stories of takotsubo

My cardiologist wanted to send me home with a defibrillating vest due to my low EF, but I refused it, since I had not seen any ventricular arrythmias, and I was afraid that my only previous arrythmia, SVT, which looks a lot like a ventricular arrythmia, might trigger a painful defibrillation shock. Although after researching TTS on the internet, I hoped to be in the 70% or more of people with TTS who recovered completely, I told my cardiologist that at my age, I did not necessarily want to live longer being barely able to walk to the bathroom without shortness of breath. So, I also declined an MRI, as well as the defibrillating vest, and the possibility of an implantable defibrillator. I think that the doctors were annoyed by this. However, on my last day, a kind young female hospitalist, who introduced herself as 'brand new', sat down, held my hand, and said that she completely understood my not wanting the defibrillating vest. I was very grateful for her sympathy and understanding.

My discharge diagnosis was takotsubo cardiomyopathy with NonSTEMI heart attack. My EF had recovered to 60-65% by about four months after my TTS event, and I have gradually worked up to walking a mile on the level with no chest pain or shortness of breath and can climb one flight of stairs easily at eight months after my TTS event. In an abundance of caution, I had help around the house during the day for about four months after my event, since I live alone.

I have had two further episodes of high heart rates that required an ER visit and IV medication to normalise. The unpredictability of these recurring tachycardia events and some chest pain with activity has been a little unnerving and makes me reluctant to travel very far, especially alone as I had been doing.

Sadly, several in my TTS support group have similar stories of serious cardiac symptoms of their TTS events being ignored in the ER. However, the group has also helped me realise that there are some post TTS complications that are not easily managed and that there are a range of recovery scenarios from TTS which even many health professionals don't realise. Many think that if they have seen one or two people with TTS who recovered quickly with no problems, that everyone should. Hopefully, further research about this rare heart disorder can focus on quicker recognition and treatment of TTS in the ER setting and better prevention and management of the associated complications.

## Catherine's story

Catherine Hughes was aged 58 when she had her first TTS. She lives in the UK and owns a prom dress shop. This is her story:

It was the 5th November – Guy Fawkes night. I was closing my shop in the evening when I noticed the mediaeval house next door appeared to have started their bonfire early; there was a lot of smoke. When I looked harder I could see smoke behind the glass in the house. I went closer to investigate and could see the house owners' cars on the drive and the family dog in an outbuilding attached to the house. I rushed over and banged on the front door to try and attract the attention of the occupants. There were no flames inside the house, just smoke, so I knew not to try and open the door as the oxygen could make the flames ignite. I immediately rang the emergency services. They arrived followed by the owners of the house who had been out on a shopping trip. I walked back to my shop and immediately felt a dull ache in the centre of my chest. I actually joked with another shop owner that I felt like I was having a heart attack.

I drove home, then cooked a family dinner, all the time the pain getting worse and travelling up to my neck. It was late evening and I was getting concerned; I didn't tell my family how I was feeling as I thought it was just shock from what had happened. I phoned the non-emergency helpline 111; they quickly realised that I needed help. An ambulance was called and once in hospital tests were carried out where they discovered raised troponin levels.

The doctors told me the next day that I had had a heart attack and would send me to another hospital to have an angiogram; this showed no blockages but an EF of 35%. They then said I had had a TTS event.

I had two years of fatigue, thinking that this was now how my life was going to be, then I started to feel normal again. Back to everything I used to do before... until the second event in 2018.

At this time I was 63 and very active; I was a keen gardener and played badminton regularly.

It was 18th March 2018 at 9:30 am. I had to tell my daughter that her partner was cheating on her. Two hours later I started to feel ill. During the day the pain came and went and at 9:15 pm I decided to go to A&E.

I told the receptionist that I was having a heart attack (I thought if I said takotsubo that she wouldn't know what I was talking about). I explained that the pain was severe and like a tight band around my chest and I had upper back pain. After an ECG, I was told there was nothing significant and that I was probably suffering from angina. I explained that I had had a takotsubo event six years earlier and that last time the ECG didn't show any signs of a heart attack and that they should still be treating me as a heart attack patient. I told the nurse that my angiogram in 2011 showed no blockages and I did not have any stents fitted.

I was given co-dydramol and moved out of Resusc into a bay in the general A&E area, and then waited in agony for almost four hours. The pain had escalated and now was severe, coming in waves mid to off-centre of the upper abdomen. At this point I buzzed for a nurse and told her that the pain was worse. She said that I was being monitored and that nothing had shown on the ECG and that they were not concerned but there would still be at least another hour until I saw a doctor.

I said to the nurse that if I had to wait another hour then I wanted blood tests done immediately, so that when the doctor eventually came to see me that the first set of blood test results would be back for the doctor to see. The blood tests came back raised at a troponin reading of 277. The doctor said I had had a heart attack but later a different doctor said that I hadn't had a heart attack and they would be probably be sending me home. I asked why when the level was reading at 277? He said it was probably high due to my previous event in 2011. I did not realise until later that these levels return to near zero within 14 days of an attack, otherwise I would have 'stood my ground'.

The next morning, the pain became unbearable and I pressed my call button. I waited for a while and no one came. A cleaner came into my cubicle and I asked her to fetch a nurse. No-one came. I called a passing doctor and then a passing nurse and still no-one came. I shouted loudly for someone to come and see me immediately. A ward sister came to see me. She said, 'What's the matter with you?' I said, 'I need someone to be with me whilst this pain is happening'. She said, 'We are too busy to sit with individual patients'. I said I didn't want someone to sit with me I just wanted someone to be with me until this episode subsided. She left and I was alone until 11:30 am when my daughter arrived. I told her I was in extreme pain.

After a little while the pain built again and I started to feel clammy. My skin felt like it was itchy and my eyes had dots before them. My daughter noticed that I looked extremely unwell and pale. My heart rate on the monitor indicated that it had dropped to 40 bpm. Jennifer went to try and fetch someone and the sister eventually returned. She saw that my heart rate was low and asked if I had used my GTN spray. I said I hadn't. She placed the blood pressure sleeve around my arm and it read 44/32 mm Hg and the alarms sounded. She quickly lowered my back rest and told me to lie flat. She went to fetch someone and three doctors arrived. I dread to think what would have been the outcome had my daughter not been with me. I was then admitted into hospital and half an hour later I was in the medical assessment unit.

I had an angiogram four days later and this showed that my heart had been seriously damaged in five different places; 50% of the muscle had been damaged.

New research does not make me feel very positive. I was a fit 64-year-old and now I am a mess. I am so angry at the incompetence of the staff in A&E.

During those 14 hours of being in A&E, I was in excruciating pain and all this time my heart muscle was being damaged.

In retrospect, I should not have ignored my symptoms. I will call for an ambulance next time and tell my family I am in pain.

I am now 70. I have had a very emotional and stressful year. When I look back at some of the emotional times I've had it amazes me that my heart has coped so well. I am coming through this year feeling well and positive. I look after my two small grandchildren three days a week. I am still playing badminton on a weekly basis. If I start to feel anxiety coming on I find a good trick is to sit quietly and control my breathing, whereas before I would feel myself getting into a blind panic. I do worry about future TTSs but also think about the old saying 'what doesn't kill you makes you stronger'.

## Linda's story

Linda was 62 at the time of her first takotsubo event. She lives in Warwickshire in the UK. This is her story:

Prior to my first takotsubo event in 2015, I was working in a high security men's prison, facilitating courses to groups of prisoners to help them address their offending behaviour and work on their thinking skills. I loved this work, although I was aware at times after prisoner interactions that I had a lot of adrenaline in my body, which meant it was difficult to get to sleep at night. I was married with three grown-up sons and had a happy family life. I was very active, had a healthy lifestyle and enjoyed walking and gardening.

On the day of my event, In February, I had left work and was meeting with a tree surgeon in the garden at my son's house in the late afternoon. It was very cold and while I was waiting outside for him to look in his diary he took a telephone call which went on and on. I could feel myself becoming extremely irritated that he wouldn't curtail his call and just deal with my situation! However, I said nothing. Once he had gone I went back inside the house to lock up and felt a sudden, extreme pain in the centre of my back and chest.

My initial thought was that it must be heartburn. It was a really intense pain. I decided I would drive the four miles home and remember thinking on the way, 'This can't be a heart attack, I'm slim and fit and I had an angiogram a couple of years ago and they said my arteries were as clean as a whistle and I was unlikely to ever have heart disease'.

When I got home I was still in incredible pain. I didn't feel it was important enough to phone for an ambulance, so I asked my neighbour to drive me a couple of miles to our local hospital. My husband wasn't home from work.

I was quickly attended to in A&E where I had an ECG and blood was taken. I was given morphine. After about four hours the pain was subsiding, and I was admitted to the hospital. The next morning the consultant said my troponin levels were high and I had had a heart attack. I was amazed! She said they were going to send me to another hospital. An echocardiogram revealed my left ventricle was distorted due to a massive adrenaline attack and an angiogram showed that my arteries were clear. I was told it was takotsubo cardiomyopathy which mainly affects post-menopausal women.

They said they had had two cases the previous year. I had never heard of it, but I was told it was good news as I hadn't had a heart attack and that I would make a full recovery. I was sent home with a one-page handout from the British Heart Foundation and said I would be seen again in three months for an echocardiogram to check my ejection fraction.

I was bewildered by this diagnosis and how little information there was on the Internet. My GP knew very little about it. I was put on a cocktail of medication that was routinely given to those who had had a heart attack. I was extremely fatigued and breathless and could do hardly anything. It was thought the beta-blockers were making me breathless, so I came off them.

## What becomes of the broken-hearted

Any exertion gave me tightness in the chest and I limited activities to making myself a drink and going to the toilet! Having a shower and washing my hair were totally exhausting. Fortunately my husband was there to cook and look after me.

After an initial, very weary six weeks, I started to slowly recover but took the decision to take early retirement, along with my husband. I adopted a simple life with walking, gardening and family being my main interests. I had volunteered to become a mentor in a local high school but due to feeling the adrenaline in my body again I had given that up.

It was a real shock to have a second episode at the end of June 2019 at the age of 66. I had been on a walking holiday in the Yorkshire Dales with my husband. At the end of that time we went to stay with a group from our church at a conference and retreat centre in Kettlewell. After giving a short presentation to the group I was aware that my pulse had shot up from a usual 40-50 bpm to 100. I suddenly experienced incredible chest pain and said to my husband to call an ambulance.

Due to the distance involved and the fact that there was a cycling event in the Dales that day, they took the decision to send for the air ambulance and I was airlifted to a hospital in Middlesborough where I stayed for four days. I remember being so disappointed that I was not even well enough to enjoy the views from the helicopter! My husband followed by car and then spent four nights in the Premier Inn.

The whole episode was being filmed for a TV programme about air ambulances. During the journey in the helicopter I was very sick with the morphine they had given me for the pain. The doctor asked if I knew what was causing the pain and told me it was caused by a clot in the heart. I hadn't got the energy to tell him that in fact a takotsubo mimics a heart attack and my arteries were clear.

I felt very ill but received excellent care from the cardiology team where they carried out the same procedures as previously to confirm it was a second takotsubo. I then returned home to Warwickshire where my husband once again looked after me as I felt unable to do anything except rest.

Soon after coming home I felt extremely unwell and was admitted to my local hospital for three days after I experienced something like a tight band around my rib cage and severe breathlessness, thought to be due to the medication I was on. Once again the beta-blockers were stopped and after 10 weeks I felt able to start cardio rehab with the physio department at the local hospital which enabled me to slowly build my fitness levels in a safe place.

I felt that my recovery took longer but I ensured I did all I could to reduce my adrenaline levels and rested well, listened to relaxation/meditation for an hour daily, walked each day and learnt to accept life as it was at that moment yet looked forward to getting my strength back. Walking up inclines when out walking still made me breathless.

In September 2020, a year after my second takotsubo, I had a third event. Following a journey home from a relaxed holiday in Dartmouth I didn't feel very well. I thought it was my stomach. The following day we had a short journey to see my son and I felt unwell in the car, with atrial fibrillations. Arriving at his house, pain started in my chest and back, so we called an ambulance. I was taken to hospital in Banbury. I knew it was another takotsubo.

This time I was clued up as I had discovered a supportive Facebook group where we could share our experiences and research papers we had found. I had learnt to become my own advocate. I said no to the beta-blockers as they shouldn't be given to people with bradycardia! On the previous two occasions I had had morphine for the pain which knocked me out for days, so this time I wanted just paracetamol. The pain wasn't as intense as the first two but was still with me for eight hours.

Initially the doctors didn't think it was a takotsubo. A few hours later a doctor came to see me and said, 'You are right'. An echocardiogram and high troponin levels confirmed takotsubo. The last time I had had an angiogram in Middlesbrough the doctor had said, 'If you ever get this again, tell them you don't need another angiogram, your arteries are clear!' They did not do one this time.

Since my third takotsubo I have been given a pacemaker due to bradycardia (low pulse) and three years later I'm generally feeling well and I've worked on increasing my stamina.

If I could share what I have learned with others going through it, I would say I have totally reassessed my lifestyle. I did not go down the anti-anxiety medication route as I wanted to try a more natural approach. I have learnt to change some of the ways I respond to situations. I have worked at reducing the fight-or-flight response (sympathetic nervous system) and activating the rest-and-digest response (parasympathetic nervous system). I now practise abdominal breathing to stimulate the vagus nerve along with meditation, mindfulness, walking in nature and limiting stressful interactions.

I am aware that not all cases of takotsubo are caused by stressful situations; some can be physical and for others there is no known cause. I would like to think that my medical information can be used to inform research, but I am not sure this happens.

## Sabine's story

Sabine Heldenmaier lives in the small town of Aalen, Germany. She was 54 at the time of her TTS event. This is her story:

My event was in September 2018. I'd had a lot of emotional stress with my husband's son, whose mother had died in 1999. My husband and I married in 2003 when his son was eight years old.

I did everything for my stepson but there was a lot of tension with his grandmother, and with my husband. The situation was not easy for the whole family and especially for me. In August 2018 there was a very bad fight between my stepson and me. This was very emotional and sad for me.

A few days later I had a pre-arranged consultation in the hospital for vascular malformation, a pre-existing condition.

After this meeting I didn't feel good; my breathing was laboured and I had nausea. I had a cardiac arrest (which was caused by TTS). Luckily I was still at the hospital when it happened. The emergency team worked for 45 minutes on resuscitation; they told my husband after 40 minutes that they had five more minutes to bring me back to life. They managed to bring me back, but I then fell into a coma for three weeks. They told me and my family that this was very rare.

TTS changed my life completely, for me and my family. My heart is still working but nothing in my life is the same as before TTS. Because of the 45 minutes' reanimation I still have physical limitation but I'm here and I have learned to live with it. Twice a year I go to the cardiologist and have a check-up of my implanted defibrillator and that's it. In five years they have changed my defibrillator but nobody has shown any interest in how I feel; they look at the physical things and the emotional things are not that important.

It took three years to regain a normal life, but with the help of my family and my little dog (a present from my husband), I did it. I'm very happy to be still alive and have joy and fun with my family, my dog and grandson.

In Germany, it is not easy to find people who have had TTS, or specialised doctors. Sometimes I feel very alone with my TTS.

## Heather's story

Heather Godfrey lives in West Sussex, UK. She is aged 75. She is a retired care worker. This is her story:

In 2017 I was diagnosed with angina and prescribed meds plus a GTN (glyceryl trinitrate) spray. (This can relieve symptoms of chest pain (angina). It quickly widens your blood vessels, increasing the blood flow to the heart.)

In August 2018, I accompanied my 15-year-old granddaughter to South Africa on an overnight flight to visit her father (as ruled in a divorce agreement). On arrival in SA, our suitcases went missing for our connecting flight. We were to-ing and fro-ing from one terminal to the other; by the time we found the luggage it was too late to board the flight.

There was more to-ing and fro-ing to change our bookings to the next flight, only to be told that was not permitted! We were also told that as we'd missed our flight, our return to UK flights would be cancelled. Stress through the roof, as you can imagine. We returned to the internal flight terminal and managed to get seats on the next flight.

We had just got through hand luggage x-ray, when I had severe chest pain; it was hard to breathe; my granddaughter got my GTN spray as I thought I was having a full-blown angina attack, but I passed out before using it. I hit the floor very hard.

I came to soon after and was helped into a wheelchair, and asked if I wanted an ambulance but said no, I would be fine. I could not leave my young granddaughter alone in Johannesburg – so we continued onto the next flight. During the two hour flight I became progressively worse; I was struggling to breathe; the GTN spray did not work. I was vomiting, the chest pain was excruciating and I was not fully aware of what was happening.

They asked for a doctor or nurse on board but there was none. Other passengers helped as much as they could and my granddaughter was an absolute star. The pilot radioed for an ambulance to meet the plane and spoke to my son and ex-son-in-law. I was very much out of it by then; paramedics had to attend to me twice on the way to hospital I was told.

At A&E, the cardiologist said it was not a stroke; they immediately rushed me to theatre as he said it was a different heart problem. An angiogram confirmed it was takotsubo and was stress related. The doctor had dealt with takotsubo before. I was prescribed: furosemide, spironalactone, omeprazole, aspirin and perindopril. I came off all except the perindopril after 18 months.

After five days in hospital I spent four days at my son's home, sleeping mostly; I just could not keep awake, but was lovingly looked after by family and friends.

Travel insurance flew me, my granddaughter and a flight doctor first class back to Johannesburg, then on to Heathrow where we were met by car ambulance, and driven home to East Grinstead. The flight doctor spent a long time telling my daughter about takotsubo and all the follow-up procedures for my GP to put in place.

The doctors at my surgery had not dealt with a takotsubo patient before.

I did return to swimming and walking, then COVID hit. I unfortunately ate through lockdowns and put on a lot of weight. I am now not able to swim; both my knees have bad meniscus tears from years of manually lifting my disabled husband. I am walking but not as much as previously... painfully!

I am having dental work done at the end of November – stressful! Local anaesthetic without adrenaline – it is quite terrifying! Other than that, I am fine, thankfully.

## Carmel's story

Carmel Lynam is 66 years old and lives in Castletown Geoghegan in Ireland. She is a retired primary school teacher. This is her story:

My cholesterol has been above the normal range for a long time now; probably 16 years. However, this is a familial problem. I have been put on Lipitor and other statins for this over the years but at this time, following my own reading up on the whole statin debate, I am taking no medication... rather I'm trying to follow a Mediterranean diet.

## Stories of takotsubo

I got my first COVID-19 (Astra Zeneka) vaccine on 10th May 2021. I was in perfect form and in perfect health prior to this. I enjoyed cycling, walking and playing pickleball with a local Active Retirement Group.

I felt perfectly well that evening and the following morning. I don't think I even had a sore arm.

I went to my local town to have my eyes tested the following day. I happened to bump into an old teaching colleague whom I hadn't spoken to since long before COVID. After my eye test we sat together having coffee and a salad roll (outdoors, COVID style!).

Very soon I began to feel an uncomfortable pain in my chest. I actually thought it was indigestion. We chatted for about a half hour and as we said goodbye I said I was going to get Gaviscon in Boots to deal with my indigestion.

After taking the Gaviscon there was no improvement whatsoever in the pain and I knew I was not well enough to get in my car. I sat on a chair in Boots. The pharmacist saw me and enquired if I was OK. I told her about my chest discomfort and she took me into a room where she took my blood pressure. I began to feel sick and a bit faint. The pharmacist took the decision to ring for an ambulance. (I actually thought she was overreacting.)

The paramedic in the ambulance did an ECG. He knew from that that there had been an event of some kind and he phoned ahead to University Hospital Galway. The pain eased somewhat on the journey though I had two further bouts of nausea and feeling faint. There was a team ready to receive me in the hospital and they did an angiogram and blood tests straight away. The angiogram showed no sign of blockage but the troponin levels in my blood were at 1500. An echocardiogram the next day showed ballooning of my left ventricle and so I was diagnosed with takotsubo.

I was shocked to hear this. I had never heard of it before and of course went to Dr Google to get all the information I could.

I was kept in hospital for almost a week and was well looked after and monitored. Apart from daily ECG, blood pressure etc, I can't remember any other tests.

Back home I felt very fatigued the whole time. My movements and even my brain function were slow. I am very fortunate in that my family and friends were very supportive and understanding.

I was put on a beta-blocker and other medications. One of these medications was reduced while I was still in hospital as it was causing my blood pressure and my heart rate to drop to a concerning level. I had regular check-ups with my cardiologist after my discharge. My medications were gradually reduced and then discontinued.

I was very uncertain when it came to getting my second vaccine but felt I had no option but to take it. If I didn't get the second vaccination then I wouldn't get my COVID certificates and consequently would not be able to travel. However, when I presented myself for the Pfizer vaccine the nurse wouldn't give it to me after I told her about my adverse reaction to the first one. I was advised to discuss it with my doctor. My doctor then referred me back to the cardiologist for his professional advice. He told me it was a decision I would have to make myself as he could not say for sure if the vaccine was the cause of my takotsubo.

As already stated I felt I had no option but to proceed with the vaccination. This time, fortunately, I had no ill effects.

I have to say that both my doctor and my cardiologist were knowledgeable on the subject of takotsubo though I have met several in the medical profession who have never heard of it.

I have had to have dental implants placed over the last few years and fortunately I had read in the takotsubo Facebook group about the importance of letting the dentist know not to use adrenaline in the anaesthetic. The dentist had no knowledge of takotsubo either.

I was feeling well recovered this year, so much so that I embarked on a cycle along the Wild Atlantic Way in June with some friends. There were some severe hills en route, especially near the Cliffs of Moher. I think now I may have put more pressure on my heart than was wise as I began to feel fatigued and breathless for a while after.

About two months later I took part in what's known locally as the Lilliput Legend. I did the cycling part (21 km) of the triathlon. Once again I didn't feel 100% for a few weeks afterwards. My blood pressure currently is much higher than it used to be: around 150 over 75 where it used to be 110 over 65 or thereabouts. I suspect it's because of the strain I put on my heart during the above activities (my own diagnosis entirely!).

I have decided that from now on any exercise I do will be more moderate. Maybe this could be termed good advice for others.

What becomes of the broken-hearted

# PART III

# Looking after your heart health

# Chapter Fifteen

# **Heart-healthy recipes**

Eating a heart-healthy diet helps to improve cholesterol levels, manage blood pressure, control blood sugar and manage weight. In this Chapter you will find a few ideas and recipes to hopefully give you some inspiration.

The goal is to limit the amount of work your heart has to do, and if you are eating a diet high in sodium or saturated fats, then your heart will need to work harder to stay healthy. The following recipes limit saturated fats, sodium and processed foods – all essential in keeping that heart strong.

# BREAKFAST

## Tofu scramble with spinach

### Ingredients (serves four)

- 15 g/1 tbsp olive oil
- 32 g/2 tbsp chopped shallot
- 450 g/1 x 16 oz package extra-firm tofu, drained and crumbled
- 3.5 g /1 tbsp nutritional yeast
- 2.3 g/1 tsp onion powder
- 1.2 g/½ tsp garlic powder
- 0.5 g/¼ tsp ground turmeric
- 0.5 g/¼ tsp ground pepper
- 0.5 g/¼ tsp salt, divided
- 30 g/1 packed cup torn fresh spinach
- 30 ml/2 tbsp unsweetened almond milk, or milk of your choice
- 2.5ml/½ tsp rice vinegar
- 1 red pepper, crushed (optional)

### Method

1. Heat the oil in a large non-stick skillet over a medium heat. Add the shallot; cook, stirring constantly, until slightly softened, about 1 minute.
2. Add the tofu; cook, stirring often, until most of the moisture has evaporated, 5 to 7 minutes. Stir in the nutritional yeast, onion powder, garlic powder, turmeric, pepper and a dash of salt; cook, stirring constantly, until the tofu is completely dry, 3 to 4 minutes.
3. Add the spinach, almond milk and vinegar to the tofu mixture. Cook, stirring occasionally, until the spinach has wilted, about 3 minutes. Sprinkle with crushed red pepper and the remaining salt.

## Wholegrain toast with cashew butter and banana-cinnamon

### Ingredients (serves one)

- 1 slice wholegrain bread, toasted
- 15 g/1 tbsp cashew butter
- 1 small banana, sliced
- Cinnamon, to taste

### Method

1. Spread the toast with the cashew butter and top with banana slices.
2. Sprinkle with cinnamon to taste.

## Chia seed pudding with fruit

### Ingredients (serves one)

- 62 g/¼ cup Greek yogurt or kefir
- 62 g/¼ cup milk of choice
- 30 g/2 tbsp chia seeds
- 10.5 g/½ tbsp honey or maple syrup
- Vanilla extract (optional)
- Dash cinnamon (optional)

## Method

1. Mix all the ingredients together until well combined.
2. Leave in the fridge overnight or for at least 2 hours.
3. Top with any or all of these: strawberries, blueberries, banana slices, nuts, coconut flakes, sprinkling of cocoa powder.

## Protein-packed pancakes

### Ingredients (for four pancakes)

- 90 g/1 cup rolled oats
- 10.8 g/2¼ tsp baking powder
- 30 g/¼ cup protein powder
- 3 small eggs
- 85 g/⅓ cup Greek yogurt
- 1.2 ml/¼ tsp vanilla extract
- 15 ml/1 tbsp maple syrup
- 15 g/1 tbsp coconut oil

### Method

1. Blend the oats in a blender or food processor until the mixture becomes like the texture of flour. Add the remaining ingredients and blend until smooth.
2. Add the oil to a non-stick pan and place over a medium-high heat.
3. When the fat is hot, drop ¼ cup portions of the batter onto the pan. Cook each pancake until bubbles appear on the surface. Lift and flip the pancake and cook for another minute.
4. Repeat the process until all the pancakes are cooked.

# Healthy burrito wrap

## Ingredients (serves four)

- 4 whole-grain wraps
- 5 large eggs
- 60 ml/¼ cup water or low-fat milk
- 30 g/2 tbsp olive oil
- 32 g/¼ cup onion or scallion, chopped
- ½ red pepper, chopped
- 44 g/½ cup mushrooms, sliced
- 60 g/2 cups baby spinach
- Dash salt and dash black pepper
- 58 g/4 tbsp Cheddar or feta cheese
- 63.5 g/¼ cup salsa

## Instructions

1. Heat a frying pan over a medium heat. Add the oil, onion, pepper and mushrooms; cook for about 3-5 minutes until the veggies are soft. Add the spinach and cook just until wilted.
2. Meanwhile, whisk the eggs together with water or milk and season with salt and pepper.
3. Pour the egg mixture into the pan and lightly scramble until it is no longer runny.
4. Warm the wraps in a microwave for 10-15 seconds or for 5 minutes under a low grill.
5. Divide the eggs between the 4 wraps.
6. Sprinkle each burrito with 1 tbsp cheese and salsa.
7. Wrap it up!

## Berry smoothie

### Ingredients (serves 1)

- 355 ml/1½ cups milk of your choice
- 1 banana, sliced
- 150 g/1½ cups frozen mixed berries
- 186 g/¾ cup vanilla Greek yogurt
- 15 g/1 tbsp honey or maple syrup, optional
- Optional garnish: fresh berries and mint sprigs

### Method

1. Place the milk, banana, berries and yogurt in a blender; blend until smooth. Add more liquid if the smoothie is too thick.
2. Taste and add honey or maple syrup if desired.
3. Garnish if desired.

## Other ideas

- Avocado on wholewheat toast
- Oatmeal with fruit
- Greek yogurt with fruit, topped with nuts and seeds and a drizzle of honey if desired
- Scrambled eggs with spinach and sliced fresh tomatoes
- Poached eggs on wholewheat toast
- Cashew butter on wholewheat toast
- Low-fat muesli with Greek yogurt, topped with flax and hemp seeds
- Wholegrain English muffin with melted cheese and sautéed mushrooms

# LUNCH

## Chickpea salad

### Ingredients (serves 4)

- 30 g/2 tbsp olive oil
- 30 ml/2 tbsp fresh lemon juice
- 1 garlic clove, grated
- 5 g/1 tsp Dijon mustard
- 5 g/1 tsp sea salt
- 510 g/3 cups cooked chickpeas, drained and rinsed
- 298 g/2 cups mixed yellow and red grape-tomatoes, halved
- ½ English cucumber, diced
- 90 g/½ cup kalamata olives, pitted and halved, optional
- 30 g/½ cup chopped fresh parsley
- 15 g/¼ cup fresh dill, chopped
- 15 g/¼ cup chopped fresh mint, plus whole mint leaves for garnish
- Freshly ground black pepper

### Method

1. In a large bowl, whisk together the olive oil, lemon juice, garlic, mustard, salt and several grinds of the pepper.
2. Add the chickpeas, tomatoes, cucumber and olives, and toss to coat. Add the parsley, dill and mint, and toss again.
3. Season to taste, garnish with fresh mint leaves, and serve.

## Mediterranean tuna salad

### Ingredients (serves 2-4)

- 1 red bell pepper, finely diced
- 1 small shallot, minced
- ½ English cucumber, chopped
- 2 x 142-g/2 x 5-oz cans white meat tuna
- 22.5 g/3 tbsp capers, drained
- 30 ml/2 tbsp white wine vinegar
- 15 g/1 tbsp olive oil
- 15 g/1 tbsp Dijon mustard
- 1.5 g/¼ tsp salt
- 30 g/2 tbsp feta cheese crumbles (optional)

### Method

1. Drain the tuna and place it in a medium bowl: mash it lightly with a fork.
2. Add the chopped vegetables, capers, white wine vinegar, olive oil, Dijon mustard, feta (if using) and salt; stir to combine. Taste and add more salt if desired.
3. Serve on its own, in a sandwich using wholegrain bread, or in a wrap.

# Curry lentil soup

## Ingredients (serves 4)

- 30 g/2 tbsp olive oil
- 1 large onion, chopped
- 2 carrots, sliced into discs
- 3 garlic cloves, grated
- 2 g/1 tsp ginger, grated
- 4 g/2 tsp curry powder
- 2 g/1 tsp turmeric powder
- 2 g/1 tsp ground cumin
- 1.2 g/½ tsp red pepper flakes – more to taste
- 1.1-4 l/5-6 cups vegetable broth
- 15 oz (1 can) crushed tomatoes
- 210 g/1 cup dry lentils, green or brown
- 454 g/1 lb potatoes, peeled and cut into bite-size chunks
- 141 g/5 oz kale or spinach, chopped
- 6 g/1 tsp salt – more to taste
- 6 g/1 tsp black pepper
- Cilantro/coriander for garnish
- 1 lime (optional) to squeeze on top

## Method

1. Heat a large pot over a medium heat. Once hot, add the oil and onion. Sauté for 3 minutes, stirring frequently, until softened and slightly browned.
2. Add the carrots and garlic and sauté for 2-3 minutes. Add salt, and stir. Cook for 1-2 minutes more, stirring occasionally.
3. Add the curry powder, turmeric, ground cumin and red pepper flakes, mix everything together, then add the vegetable broth and increase the heat from medium to high. Bring to a low boil.

4. Add the tomatoes, lentils and potatoes and stir. Bring back to a low boil, then reduce the heat to low or until you achieve a gentle simmer.
5. Simmer the soup uncovered, stirring occasionally, for 15-20 minutes or until the carrots and lentils are tender (red lentils cook pretty quickly, so if you're using other lentils, adjust the cook time as needed).
6. If the mixture becomes too thick, you can add more vegetable broth as needed.
7. Add the kale or spinach for the last 5 minutes of cooking.
8. Divide between serving bowls, sprinkle with salt and pepper and garnish with fresh cilantro/coriander and a squeeze of lime juice.

## Mexican-style baked sweet potatoes

### Ingredients (serves 2)

- 2 medium sweet potatoes
- 172 g/1 cup black beans
- 90 g/½ cup sweetcorn, drained
- ½ avocado, diced
- 8 cherry tomatoes, cut in half
- ¼ red onion, finely diced
- ¼ tsp salt
- 15 ml/1 tbsp lime juice, divided
- 89 g/1 cup red cabbage, shredded
- Handful broccoli sprouts

### For yogurt cilantro/coriander sauce
- 125 g/½ cup yogurt
- ½ jalapeño
- 17 g/½ cup cilantro/coriander
- 30 g/2 tbsp hemp seeds
- 2 g/1 tsp cumin
- 15 ml/1 tbsp lime juice

## *Method*

1. Preheat your oven to 200°C/400°F.
2. Slice the sweet potatoes in half lengthways. Place them on a parchment-lined baking tray, face down.
3. Bake for 45 minutes, until tender.
4. While the potatoes are baking, prepare the filling. Mix together in a bowl the black beans, corn, avocado, cherry tomatoes, red onion, salt and half of the lime juice.
5. In a separate bowl, massage the red cabbage with the remaining lime juice until it turns bright pink.
6. For the sauce, blend the yogurt, jalapeño, lime juice, coriander, hemp seeds and cumin until smooth.
7. Once the sweet potatoes are baked, flip them over and gently mash the insides with a fork.
8. Top the sweet potatoes with the black bean mixture, cabbage and broccoli sprouts.
9. Drizzle with the sauce and serve.

## Chopped cobb salad with chicken

### Ingredients

- 95 g/2 cups chopped romaine lettuce
- 50 g/¼ cup chopped tomato
- 44 g/¼ cup chopped cucumber
- 30 g/¼ cup sliced white button mushrooms
- 85 g/3 oz grilled or roasted chicken breast, cut into cubes or strips
- 2 hard-boiled eggs, chopped
- 60 g/¼ cup no-salt-added cannellini beans, drained and rinsed

### For the dressing

- 53 g/¼ cup olive oil
- 30 ml/2 tbsp balsamic vinegar, or lemon juice, or apple cider vinegar
- 15-30 g/1-2 tbsp mustard of choice
- 1 clove garlic, crushed

### Method

1. Make the dressing: whisk all the dressing ingredients together in a small jar or bowl.
2. Place the lettuce in a medium bowl and add 1 tbsp of the dressing; toss to coat.
3. Arrange the tomato, cucumber, mushrooms, chicken, egg and beans in rows on top of the lettuce. Drizzle with the remaining dressing.

## Mason-jar power salad with chickpeas and tuna

### Ingredients (serves 1)

- 67 g/1 cup bite-sized pieces chopped kale
- 30 g/2 tbsp honey-mustard vinaigrette (see recipe on page 184)
- 56 g/¼ cup tuna (canned in water)
- 85 g/½ cup chickpeas (canned), rinsed and drained
- 1 carrot, peeled and shredded

### Method

1. Toss the kale and dressing in a bowl, then transfer to a mason jar.
2. Top with the tuna, chickpeas and carrot.
3. Screw the lid onto the jar and refrigerate for up to 2 days.
4. To serve, empty the jar contents into a bowl and toss to combine the salad ingredients with the dressed kale.

## Honey mustard vinaigrette

### Ingredients

- 1 clove garlic, minced
- 15 ml/1 tbsp white-wine vinegar
- 10 g/1½ tsp Dijon mustard (coarse or smooth)
- 3.5 g/½ tsp honey
- Pinch of salt
- Freshly ground pepper, to taste
- 71 g/⅓ cup extra-virgin olive oil, or avocado oil

### Method

1. Whisk the garlic, vinegar, mustard, honey, salt and pepper in a small bowl.
2. Slowly whisk in the oil.

## Creamy sweet potato soup

### Ingredients (serves 4)

- 700 g/1½ lb sweet potatoes
- 230 g/½ lb carrots, chopped
- 1 medium onion, chopped
- 3 cloves garlic, grated
- 15 g/1 tbsp extra-virgin olive oil
- 2½ cm/1 inch fresh ginger, grated
- Pinch red pepper flakes
- 4 g/1 tsp ground cumin
- 3 g/½ tsp salt
- 2.5 g/½ tsp black pepper
- 1½ l/5-6 cups of vegetable broth; add more or less depending on

## Heart-healthy recipes

- your preferred consistency
- 1 large apple, peeled and diced
- 400 g/14 oz can coconut milk
- Cilantro/coriander for serving

## **Method**

1. Heat the olive oil in a large pot or Dutch oven.
2. Add the onion and carrots, fry for 3 minutes, then add the garlic and ginger, cumin, pinch of red pepper flakes, and fry for another minute.
3. Add the vegetable broth, sweet potatoes and apple, salt and pepper.
4. Cover with a lid, bring to the boil and then simmer (with the lid cracked) for around 20 minutes, until the potatoes are tender.
5. Turn off the heat and blend with an immersion blender until smooth.
6. Stir in the coconut milk, and simmer for 5 more minutes.
7. Taste, and adjust seasoning accordingly.
8. Serve with the squeezed lime juice, sprinkling of cilantro/coriander and a few red pepper flakes if desired.

## Chicken and cucumber lettuce wraps with peanut sauce

### Ingredients (serves 4)

- 65 g/¼ cup creamy peanut butter
- 30 ml/2 tbsp low-sodium soy sauce
- 42 g/2 tbsp honey
- 30 ml/2 tbsp water
- 10 g/2 tsp toasted sesame oil
- 10 g/2 tsp olive oil
- 3 scallions, sliced, white and green parts separated
- 1 serrano pepper, seeded and minced (2 tsp)
- 7 g/1 tbsp minced fresh ginger
- 6 g/2 tsp minced fresh garlic
- 453 g/1 lb ground chicken breast
- 16 butter lettuce leaves
- 195 g/1 cup cooked brown rice
- 126 g/1 cup halved and thinly sliced English cucumber
- 25 g/½ cup fresh cilantro/coriander leaves
- Lime wedges, for serving

### Method

1. To make the peanut sauce, whisk the peanut butter, soy sauce, honey, water and sesame oil together in a small bowl.
2. Heat the olive oil in a large non-stick skillet over a medium heat. Add the scallion whites, serrano, ginger and garlic; cook until starting to soften – about 2 minutes.
3. Add the chicken and cook it, breaking it up with a spoon or potato masher, until cooked through – 3 to 4 minutes.
4. Add the peanut sauce to the chicken mixture; cook until the sauce has thickened – about 3 minutes.
5. Remove from the heat and stir in the scallion greens.

6. To serve, make 8 stacks of 2 lettuce leaves each. Divide the rice, chicken mixture, cucumber, and cilantro/coriander among the lettuce cups. Serve with the lime wedges.

## Other lunch ideas

### Wholegrain sandwiches filled with:

- Hummus with veggies – cucumber, tomatoes, lettuce, onions
- Egg and salad
- Tuna and cucumber
- Chicken breast with lettuce
- Cashew butter and banana

### Wholegrain wraps filled with:

- Tuna and sweetcorn with a slight dash of mayo
- Grilled chicken, cucumber, tomatoes and honey-mustard vinaigrette
- Boiled eggs, mashed, with bean sprouts and cucumbers
- Hummus, tomatoes, cucumber and lettuce

### Baked sweet potatoes filled with:

- Tuna and sweetcorn
- Low-fat cheese with 2 tbsp baked beans
- Mixed salad with chopped boiled eggs and avocado
- Mix kale, red onion and rocket together with feta cheese and pumpkin seeds
- Veggie chilli (see page 188) topped with avocado and cilantro/coriander.

# DINNER

## Easy veggie chilli

### Ingredients (serves 4)

- 500 ml/2 cups (3 medium) fresh tomatoes, diced
- 250 ml/1 cup canned navy beans, drained and rinsed
- 1 small can (156 ml/5.5 oz) tomato paste
- 175 g/1 cup frozen corn
- 1 can (540 ml/19 oz) chickpeas, drained and rinsed
- 1 red pepper, diced
- 1 green pepper, diced
- 5 g/1 tsp onion powder
- 5 g/1 tsp garlic powder
- 10 g/2 tsp chili powder
- 60 g/¼ cup grated light cheddar cheese
- 1 green onion, sliced

### Method

1. Purée the tomatoes, navy beans and tomato paste in a food processor, then transfer the mixture to a large stock pot.
2. Add the rest of the ingredients and simmer over a medium heat for 20 to 25 minutes, stirring occasionally.
3. Divide between 4 bowls and top with a sprinkle of the cheese and green onions.

## Sheet-pan cashew chicken

### Ingredients (serves 3)

- 3 boneless, skinless chicken breasts, cut into 1 inch/2.5 cm pieces
- 180 g/2 cups broccoli florets
- 1 red bell pepper, diced
- 120 g/1 cup unsalted cashews
- Cilantro/coriander, lime wedges for serving

**For the sauce**
- 43 g/3 tbsp siracha
- 30 ml/2 tbsp gluten-free soy sauce
- 30 ml/2 tbsp rice vinegar
- 30 ml/2 tbsp sesame oil
- 21 g/1 tbsp honey
- 2 garlic cloves, minced
- 2.5 cm/1 inch fresh ginger, peeled and minced

### Method

1. Preheat your oven to 200°C/400°F.
2. Line a large baking sheet with parchment paper.
3. Add the chicken, broccoli, pepper and cashews to the baking sheet.
4. Mix together the ingredients for the sauce in a small bowl.
5. Pour three-quarters of the sauce on the chicken and veggies, and toss to coat evenly.
6. Roast for 25 minutes, tossing halfway through.
7. Top the chicken and veggies with the remaining sauce, and toss again.
8. Serve with rice if desired, plus the cilantro/coriander, and a squeeze of lime juice.

## Grilled chicken barley bowl

### Ingredients (serves 4)

- 125 ml/½ cup pearl or pot barley
- 500 g/2 cups baby arugula
- 4 carrots, sliced lengthwise
- 2 red peppers, quartered
- 2 boneless, skinless chicken breasts (around 454 g/1 lb)
- 12 ml/2 tsp olive oil, divided
- 5 g/1 tsp chilli powder
- 10 ml/2 tsp balsamic vinegar

### Method

1. In a small saucepan, cover the barley with water and bring to a boil. Reduce the heat and simmer for around 20 minutes or until the barley is tender. Drain well.
2. Toss with the arugula and set aside.
3. Spray the carrots and peppers with olive or avocado oil cooking spray; set them aside.
4. Toss the chicken breasts with 1 tsp (5 ml) of the oil and coat them with the chilli powder.
5. Heat your grill to a medium-high heat and grill the carrots, peppers and chicken breasts – 7-8 minutes for the vegetables, 12-14 minutes for the chicken.
6. Turn occasionally until the vegetables are tender and chicken is no longer pink inside. Remove the chicken to a chopping board.
7. Slice the carrots and peppers; toss them with remaining oil and vinegar.
8. Divide the barley mixture among 4 bowls and top with the vegetables.
9. Slice the chicken and place the slices over the top to serve.

# Kale, ginger and sweet potato stew with lentils and coconut milk

## Ingredients (serves 4)

- 15 g/1 tbsp olive oil or coconut oil
- 1 medium onion, diced
- 5 g/1 tsp dried chilli flakes
- 2.5 g/½ tsp ground coriander
- 2.5 g/½ tsp ground turmeric
- 2.5 g/½ tsp ground cumin
- 1 inch/2.5 cm piece of fresh ginger, peeled and minced
- 3 cloves garlic, peeled and minced
- Sea salt and black pepper
- 690 g/1½ lb sweet potatoes, peeled and diced into 1 inch/2.5 cm pieces
- 100 g/½ cup brown lentils
- 710 ml/3 cups vegetable stock
- 400 ml/13.5 oz can full fat coconut milk
- 1 small bunch kale (approx. 90 g/4 cups chopped kale), stems removed and leaves finely chopped
- Garnish: chopped cilantro/coriander, extra chilli flakes, lime wedges

## Method

1. Heat a heavy-bottomed pot over a medium heat and add the coconut or olive oil to the pot.
2. Add the onions and sauté them, stirring occasionally, until translucent – approximately 5 minutes.
3. Add the chilli flakes, cumin, coriander and turmeric. Sauté the spices until fragrant – approximately 1 minute.
4. Add the garlic and ginger and cook for a further minute.
5. Add a pinch of salt and pepper.
6. Add the sweet potatoes to the pot and stir to coat the pieces in the spices.

7. Add the lentils and stir. Season with salt and pepper.
8. Add the vegetable stock and stir, scraping up any browned bits on the bottom. Place a lid on the pot and bring to the boil.
9. Once boiling, lower the heat to a simmer and place the lid on the pot slightly askew so that the steam can escape.
10. Simmer for around 30 minutes, until the lentils are tender.
11. Add the coconut milk and kale to the pot and stir.
12. Cover with the lid and continue to simmer until the kale is wilted – around 4 minutes. Season with salt and pepper.
13. Bring back to a simmer and check the seasoning. Add more salt, pepper or chilli flakes if necessary.
14. Serve hot with the chopped cilantro/coriander, chilli flakes and lime wedges.

# Healthy fish tacos

## Ingredients (serves 4)

### For the tacos
- 454 g/1 lb tilapia, halibut or other white fish, like cod or sea bass
- 1 lime, juiced
- 5 g/1 tsp garlic powder
- 5 g/1 tsp cumin
- 1 g/¼ tsp cayenne pepper
- 1 g/¼ tsp sea salt
- 8 small corn tortillas
- Lime wedges, for serving
- Hot sauce or salsa, for serving – optional

### For the honey Dijon cabbage slaw
- 90 g/1 cup red cabbage, thinly sliced
- 40 g/⅓ cup red onion, thinly sliced
- 18 g/⅓ cup cilantro/coriander, coarsely chopped
- 30 ml/2 tbsp fresh lime juice
- 6 g/1 tsp Dijon mustard
- 3 g/½ tsp honey
- 1 g/¼ tsp sea salt
- Ground pepper, to taste

### For the avocado crema
- 1 large avocado
- 65 g/¼ cup Greek yogurt
- Juice from 1½ limes – around 44 ml/3 tbsp
- 32 g/3 tbsp fresh cilantro/coriander
- 3 g/½ tsp salt
- 30 ml/2 tbsp water

## Method

1. Place the fish in a shallow dish and squeeze the juice from one lime over it.
2. In a small bowl, whisk together the garlic powder, cumin, cayenne and sea salt. Sprinkle the mixture over the fish and gently rub the seasoning in. Allow the fish to marinate for about 10 minutes.
3. Meanwhile, make the slaw. In a large bowl combine the cabbage, onion, cilantro/coriander, juice from the lime, mustard, honey, salt and pepper. Toss to combine. Set aside. Taste the slaw and season with additional salt and pepper, if desired.
4. Make the avocado crema by combining the avocado, yogurt, cilantro/coriander, lime juice, salt and water in a blender or food processor and blend until smooth and combined. Set aside.

5. Heat the grill to medium-high and lightly oil the grill-grate with cooking spray. Grill the fish until cooked through – 3 to 4 minutes per side.
6. Arrange the tortillas in a stack and wrap them with aluminum foil. Place them on a cooler part of grill until warm – 5 to 8 minutes, turning halfway. Alternatively, you can warm the tortillas in the oven and cook the fish on the stovetop over a medium-high heat with a little olive oil for about 3 minutes each side.
7. Break the fish into large pieces and divide it among the tortillas and top with the slaw and avocado crema.
8. Serve each taco with a small lime wedge to squeeze over the taco before eating.

## Healthy baked salmon

### Ingredients (serves 4)

- 4 salmon fillets – around 170 g/6 oz each
- 30 g/2 tbsp olive oil
- 1 g/¼ tsp salt
- 1 g/¼ tsp fresh black pepper
- 17 g/2 tbsp minced garlic
- 5 g/1 tsp Italian herb seasoning blend
- 1 medium lemon

### Method

1. Preheat your oven to 200°C/400°F.
2. Arrange the salmon fillets on a parchment-lined baking sheet and season generously with salt and pepper.
3. Stir together the olive oil, garlic, herbs and juice of half a lemon. Spoon this mixture over the salmon fillets and rub the mixture all over the tops and sides of the salmon.
4. Thinly slice the remaining half lemon and top each piece of salmon with a lemon slice.
5. Bake for 12-15 minutes until the salmon is opaque and flaky when pulled apart with a fork. Place under the grill for the last couple of minutes if desired.
6. Garnish with fresh thyme or parsley.

## Chickpea chicken dinner bowl

### Ingredients (serves 4)

- 3 bell peppers – any colour you like
- 150 g/¾ cup tomatoes, chopped
- 300 g/10.5 oz chicken breast
- ½ red onion
- Olive oil
- Spices: salt, pepper, chilli, garlic
- Sliced avocado
- Lettuce
- 180 g/1 cup couscous

**For crispy chickpeas**
- 400 g/1½ cups chickpeas
- 30-60 g/2-4 tbsp olive oil
- Spices: chilli powder, paprika, oregano, salt and pepper

**For the sauce:**
- 30-45 g/2-3 tbsp olive oil
- 60 g/4 tbsp plain yogurt
- 10 g/1 tsp honey
- Squeeze of fresh lemon
- Spices: dried basil, garlic, oregano, chilli, paprika, salt and pepper

## Method

1. Cut the vegetables and chicken into small cubes and place them on a parchment-lined baking tray.
2. Mix the chickpeas in the spices and place on a parchment-lined baking tray.
3. Place the chickpeas and the chicken and vegetables in the oven and bake for approximately 25-30 minutes. The chicken and veg should be tender; the chickpeas should be crispy.
4. Make the sauce: mix together the olive oil, plain yogurt, honey, lemon juice and spices and adjust as required.
5. Assemble the bowls:
    - Add a layer of lettuce and couscous to the base of the bowl.
    - Add roasted veg/chicken, then chickpeas.
    - Add some sliced avocado.
    - Drizzle with the sauce.

## Chickpea 'meat'balls with spaghetti

Using chickpeas is a great way to add fibre to your meal, and they are a great red meat alternative.

### Ingredients (serves 4)

- 400 g/2 cups chickpeas, drained
- 180 g/1 cup couscous or quinoa
- ½ red onion
- 3 garlic cloves
- 5 g/1 tsp paprika
- 10 g/2 tsp parsley
- 15 ml/1 tbsp soy sauce or tamari
- Black pepper
- Salt

**For the sauce:**
- 60 ml/4 tbsp hot sauce
- 30 ml/2 tbsp soy sauce or tamari
- 10 g/2 tsp brown sugar
- 15 g/1 tbsp cornstarch
- 30 ml/2 tbsp water

### Method

1. Preheat your oven to 200°C/400°F.
2. Place the couscous in a bowl and cover with hot water. Place a tea towel and plate over the bowl. Let is stand for 5 to 10 minutes until soft and fluffy.
3. In a food processor, add the drained chickpeas, red onion, garlic, seasonings, soy sauce and cooked couscous. Pulse until combined, but do not allow to get mushy.
4. Roll the chickpea mixture into balls using your hands, then

place on a greased baking sheet, or a layer of parchment paper.
5. Bake for 30 minutes, turning halfway, until lightly browned and crispy.
6. Serve with cooked wholewheat spaghetti – or a pasta alternative, for instance red lentil, quinoa or chickpea pasta.

# DESSERTS

## Watermelon fruit pizza

This looks and tastes amazing, trust me... and is a very healthy dessert option, especially for a dinner party.

### Ingredients (serves 4)

- 125 g/½ cup low-fat plain yogurt
- 7 g/1 tsp honey
- 1 g/¼ tsp vanilla extract
- 2 large round slices watermelon (about 1 inch/2.5 cm thick), cut from the centre of the melon – then cut each slice into 8 wedges
- 110 g/⅔ cup sliced strawberries
- 70 g/½ cup halved blackberries
- 3 kiwi fruit, sliced
- 3.5 g/2 tbsp torn fresh mint leaves

### Method

1. Combine the yogurt, honey and vanilla in a small bowl.
2. Spread 65 g/¼ cup of the yogurt mixture over each slice of watermelon.
3. Top with the strawberries, blackberries, kiwi and mint.

# Healthy chocolate mousse

## Ingredients (serves 4)

- 350 g/1½ cups plain Greek yogurt – 2% or 5% fat
- 200 g/1 cup plain (dark) chocolate chips
- 35 g/⅓ cup sifted cacao powder

## Method

1. Place the chocolate chips in a microwave-safe bowl and melt in the microwave in 30-second increments, making sure the chocolate does not burn. Repeat until fully melted. (Alternatively, melt the chocolate over a *bain marie*.)
2. Allow the chocolate to cool.
3. Add the Greek yogurt, melted chocolate and cacao powder to a bowl and mix using a hand or electric mixer. Whisk until creamy.
4. Add a few splashes of milk if you prefer your mousse a little thinner.
5. Pour into individual cups or ramekins, cover and place in the fridge for a couple of hours or overnight.
6. Add toppings of choice: delicious with raspberries, grated dark chocolate or flaky sea salt.

## Blueberry yogurt clusters

### Ingredients (serves 4)

- 410 g/2.5 cups blueberries, washed and dried
- 250 g/1 cup low-fat vanilla Greek yogurt

### Method

1. Combine the blueberries and yogurt in a bowl.
2. Spoon the mixture onto a parchment-lined plate in four clusters.
3. Freeze until set.


## Avocado chocolate pudding

### Ingredients (serves 4)

- 2 ripe avocados, pitted
- 90 ml/6 tbsp milk of your choice
- 35 g/⅓ cup sifted cacao powder
- 66 ml/5 tbsp maple syrup
- 5 ml/1 tsp vanilla extract
- Pinch salt

### Method

1. Add the avocados, milk, cocoa powder, maple syrup, vanilla extract and salt to a blender or food processor.
2. Blend until smooth and creamy, stopping as necessary to scrape down the sides. Taste and adjust for flavour.
3. Spoon the mixture into glass bowls and refrigerate until ready to serve.
4. Serve chilled with coconut whipped cream and raspberries.

# Baked apples

## Ingredients (serves 6)

- 6 medium apples
- 50 g/½ cup rolled oats
- 40 g/⅓ cup walnuts
- Pinch fine sea salt
- 17 g/2 tbsp flax seeds
- 4 g/1 tsp cinnamon
- 40 g/2 tbsp pure maple syrup

## Method

1. Preheat your oven to 200°C/400°F.
2. Wash and core the apples and place them in a glass or ceramic baking dish.
3. Place the oats, nuts, flax, cinnamon and salt in a blender or food processor and pulse until well mixed and crumbly.
4. Transfer the mixture to a small bowl. Pour in the maple syrup and stir until well combined.
5. Evenly distribute the oat and honey mixture into the apple cavities and then pour in water to a ¼ inch/0.5 cm up the side of the baking dish.
6. Bake for 45 minutes to 1 hour, or until the apples are soft. If your apples are bigger, the cooking time will be longer. Baked apples are fully cooked when you can easily stick a fork into them.
7. Serve with crème frâiche or Greek yogurt.

## Dark chocolate cashew clusters

### Ingredients (makes 24 clusters)

- 113 g/1 cup unsalted roasted cashews
- 175 g/6 oz dark chocolate chips, chopped
- Pinch flaky sea salt

### Method

1. Line a 24-cup mini-muffin tin with liners.
2. Divide the cashews among the prepared cups (about 4 cashews each).
3. Place the chocolate in a medium microwave-safe bowl; microwave on medium for 1 minute. Stir, then continue microwaving on medium in 20-second intervals until melted, stopping to stir after each interval. (Alternatively, melt the chocolate over a *bain marie*.)
4. Spoon about 1 tsp chocolate over each portion of cashews. Sprinkle evenly with salt.
5. Refrigerate until set – about 30 minutes.

# Healthy fudge brownies

## Ingredients (serves 4)

- 3 bananas
- 120 g/½ cup almond butter, or any nut butter of your choice
- 25 g/¼ cup cocoa powder
- Handful dark chocolate chips or chunks, if desired

## Method

1. Preheat your oven to 180°C/350°F.
2. Line a square baking dish with baking parchment.
3. Mash the bananas in a bowl, then add the nut butter and cocoa powder. Mix until smooth.
4. Pour the mixture into the baking tray, top with chocolate chips or chunks if desired, and bake for 18-20 mins.
5. Allow to cool before serving.

## Fruit skewers

### Ingredients (makes 4 skewers)

- 4 fresh raspberries
- 4 fresh strawberries, quartered
- 4 cubes peeled mango
- 4 pineapple chunks
- 4 peeled kiwi chunks
- 4 green grapes
- 4 red grapes
- 8 blueberries

### Method

1. Take 4 wooden skewers and thread on to each one raspberry, strawberry, mango chunk, pineapple chunk, kiwi piece, grape, and finish with 2 blueberries.
2. Serve with Greek yogurt as a dip.

# HEART-HEALTHY SNACKS

## Easy garlicky kale

### Ingredients (serves 2-4)

- 1 bunch kale
- 13 g/1 tbsp olive oil
- 3 g/1 tsp garlic, minced

### Method

1. Soak the kale leaves in a large bowl of water until dirt falls to the bottom – about 2 minutes.
2. Lift the kale from the bowl without drying the leaves and immediately remove and discard the stems.
3. Chop the kale leaves into 2.5cm (1 inch) pieces.
4. Heat the olive oil in a large pan over a medium heat; add and stir in the garlic; fry until sizzling – about 1 minute.
5. Add the kale to the pan and place a cover over the top.
6. Cook, stirring occasionally with tongs, until the kale is bright green and slightly tender – 5 to 7 minutes.

Serve as a side salad or as a snack

## Choccie blueberries

### Ingredients (serves 4)

- 380 g/2 cups fresh blueberries
- 200 g/7 oz dark chocolate, minimum 70% cocoa

### Method

1. Wash and dry the blueberries and place them in a bowl.
2. Melt the chocolate in your microwave, or over a *bain marie*.
3. Pour the melted chocolate over the blueberries and mix well until the fruit is coated.
4. Using a spoon, scoop out portions of the choccie-coated blueberries, place in clusters onto a parchment-lined plate.
5. Place in the fridge for a minimum of 1 hour.

NB: You can also use strawberries, raspberries or kiwi.

# Carrot fries

## Ingredients (serves 2-4)

- 4 carrots, sliced lengthwise
- 27-40 g/2-3 tbsp coconut or olive oil
- Seasoning:
    - 5 g/2 tsp paprika
    - 2.5 g/1 tsp onion powder
    - 5 g/2 tsp basil or oregano
    - Salt and pepper
    - 10 g/2 tbsp grated Parmesan cheese (optional)

**For the dip:**
- 82 g/⅓ cup yogurt
- 13 g/1 tbsp olive oil
- 3.5 g/½ tsp honey
- Seasoning as preferred: chilli, paprika, basil, salt and pepper

## Method

1. Preheat your oven to 180°C/350°F.
2. Cut the carrots lengthwise – in half and then half again.
3. Place in a bowl, add the oil and seasonings as required. Mix it all together.
4. Spread the carrots on a parchment-lined baking sheet – make sure they are separate.
5. Put the baking sheet into the oven and bake for around 20-30 minutes until the carrots are crispy/slightly brown.
6. Mix all the dip ingredients together and place in a small bowl.
7. Serve the carrots warm with the dip.

## Crispy smashed Brussels sprouts

### Ingredients (serves 4-6)

- 900 g/2 lb small Brussels sprouts, cleaned and trimmed
- 27 g/2 tbsp olive oil
- 15 g/¼ cup nutritional yeast
- 1 tsp salt
- 2.33 g/½ tsp ground black pepper

### Method

1. Preheat your oven to 200°C/400°F.
2. Boil or steam the sprouts until tender; drain and stir them in a bowl together with the oil and seasoning.
3. Smash them! Use a heavy-bottomed glass to press down until they are flat-ish.
4. Bake them in the oven for around 15 minutes.
5. Broil/grill them for a few minutes until golden brown.

## High-protein flaxseed bread

### Ingredients

- 270 g/2 cups ground flaxseeds
- 4 g/1 tsp baking powder
- 6 organic eggs
- 118 ml/½ cup water
- 71 g/⅓ cup coconut oil or olive oil
- Optional: add herbs or spices, for example salt, pepper, oregano

## Method

1. Preheat your oven to 180°C/350°F.
2. Line a baking tin with baking parchment.
3. Add all the ingredients to a mixing bowl, mix well, and then add the mixture to the baking tin.
4. Bake for 35-40 minutes or until the bread is firm to the touch.
5. This bread is delicious when toasted; add sliced banana and/or cashew butter for a healthy and delicious treat.

## Other snack ideas

- Handful of unsalted almonds or walnuts
- Half a cup of mixed berries
- Greek yogurt with berries
- Fresh fruit – oranges, melon, grapes, papaya, banana
- Avocado on wholegrain toast
- Celery and carrot strips
- Wholegrain rice cakes, with cashew butter if desired
- Baked or raw apples, sprinkled with cinnamon if desired
- Handful of edamame beans, with a tiny sprinkling of salt
- A few squares of dark chocolate.

# Chapter Sixteen

# About suicide

In conducting research for this book, and struggling to find conclusive, reliable facts and statistics, I have decided that I will write a book about suicide in 2025; it will focus on my own experience as a suicide-bereaved daughter; the experiences of both of my adult children – both of whom have had suicidal ideation; the exploration of the connection between ADHD and suicide; and guidance and advice from professionals. We need to know more, and we need to tackle the wall of silence that exists around this sad epidemic. In the meantime, I include below as much reliable information as I can find for readers of a book about a little-understood heart problem who will almost certainly also had a brush with suicide – in family, friends, colleagues or in their own ideation – at some time in ther lives.

In 2023, the World Health Organization (WHO) reported that more than 720,000 people die by suicide each year worldwide. That's one person every 40 seconds. Many more attempt it.

· Suicide statistics reveal that women are roughly three times more likely to attempt suicide, though men are two to four times more likely to die by suicide. Compared to men, women show higher rates of suicidal thinking, non-fatal suicidal behaviour, and suicide attempts.

The differences between attempts and completed suicides in women have erroneously led many people to believe that suicide attempts in women are often a method of getting attention rather than a serious risk. This is far from true. It's important to note that among women, an attempted (but failed) suicide attempt is the greatest risk factor for suicide in the future, and all suicide attempts, whether in men or women, need to be taken very seriously.[9]

## The risk factors

There are many risk factors, of course, but two issues that stand out particularly are ADHD and bipolar:

**ADHD:** There is a clear link between suicide ideation and ADHD. In a Canadian study published in 2020, it was found that 14% of adults with ADHD had attempted suicide, compared to 2.7% without ADHD. In the same study it was found that one in four women with ADHD had attempted suicide.[12*]

**Bipolar:** Globally, approximately 15–20% of people with bipolar disorder die by suicide, with 30–60% making at least one attempt.[13]

Among the other risk factors are clinical depression, substance use disorders and psychosis, as well as anxiety, traumatic brain injury, and personality and eating-related disorders. Situational depression can also lead to increased suicidal ideation. Often this temporary condition can be triggered by grief, relationship breakdowns, financial problems or illness, among all the other things that life throws at us.

## Suicide rate by country

Lesotho, a small country in Southern Africa, has the highest suicide rate in the world. The most recent statistics show that 87.5 people out of 100,000 die by suicide there each year.

It is more than double the next country on the list, Guyana in South America, where the figure is 40.3, and 10 times the global average of nine suicides per 100,000 people.

The countries with the lowest rates are Antigua and Barbuda, at 0.4 per 100,000, followed by Barbados at 0.6, Grenada and 0.7 and Saint Vincent and the Grenadines, at 1 per 100,000. All four countries are in the Caribbean.

## Age factor

While suicide rates have generally been falling globally, there is reportedly a rising trend of youth suicide (in the 15 to 29 year group). It is now the third leading cause of death among that age group, in over half of the countries in the world. The recorded rate in 2019 was 7.4 out of 100,000. Suicide rates were higher in males (10.5) than in females (4.1).[14]

The highest at-risk age group is the 65 and over in almost all regions of the world.

## The downward trend in suicide

It's worth noting that all suicide numbers should be taken with a hefty pinch of salt. Many countries underreport suicide deaths – due to data lags, as well as reasons related to stigma and religion. In some countries, suicide is still illegal. Nevertheless, it's worth looking at the downward trend to see what lessons it can impart.

A big chunk of that decrease can be attributed to suicide declines in the two most populous countries in the world. Between 1990 and 2016, suicide rates decreased by 15% in India and by over 60% in China. A fast-growing Chinese economy resulted in far more people moving from the countryside to more urban areas. This meant that, in addition to more economic stability, they had reduced access to pesticides, a common means of suicide in lower-income countries, especially among young women in rural areas.

Banning or limiting access to dangerous pesticides has had astonishing effects in many other Asian countries too. In 1995, Sri Lanka had the highest suicide rate in the world. The same year, it banned dangerous pesticides, and the national suicide rate has since fallen by 70%. In Bangladesh, a similar ban led to a 65% reduction. Elsewhere, means-restriction methods such as barriers on high structures, gun control laws, and smaller medication packet sizes have been shown to considerably reduce suicide rates.[16]

If you feel suicidal, please see the helplines listed on page 221 of this book.

If you know someone who is suicidal, please see below:
- When a person tells you that they are suicidal you must take them seriously.
- If you are worried that somebody is suicidal, you can ask them, if you feel comfortable doing so. Research shows that talking to someone openly about suicide does not increase their risk of suicide.
- If you are comfortable speaking with them about suicide, try to use clear and direct language – for example, 'I care a lot

about you. Do you feel suicidal?'
- People with lived experience of suicide highlight how helpful it is to have someone to talk to who listens. It is not about coming up with solutions, but about listening to the person and supporting them to explore options for seeking help and safety.
- It is important to encourage the seeking of professional support. You can help the person you are supporting by being there for them when they call a helpline or make an appointment with a health professional.
- It is also critical that you look after your own mental health and wellbeing and seek support of your own.[11]

# References

1. Assad J, Femia G, Pender P, Badie T, Rajaratnam R. Takotsubo Syndrome: A Review of Presentation, Diagnosis and Management. *Clin Med Insights Cardiol* 2022; 16: 11795468211065782. doi: 10.1177/11795468211065782. PMID: 35002350; PMCID: PMC8733363.

2. Mitchell AM, Kim Y, Prigerson HG, Mortimer MK. Complicated grief and suicidal ideation in adult survivors of suicide. *Suicide Life Threat Behav* 2005; 35: 498–506.

3. Cammann VL, Würdinger M, Ghadri JR, Templin C. Takotsubo Syndrome: Uncovering Myths and Misconceptions. *Curr Atheroscler Rep* 2021; 23(9): 53. doi: 10.1007/s11883-021-00946-z. PMID: 34268666; PMCID: PMC8282560.

4. Murakami T, Komiyama T, Kobayashi H, Ikari Y. Gender Differences in Takotsubo Syndrome. *Biology (Basel)* 2022; 11(5): 653. doi: 10.3390/biology11050653. PMID: 35625378; PMCID: PMC9138502.

5. Schweiger V, Cammann VL, Crisci G, et al. Temporal Trends in Takotsubo Syndrome: Results From the International Takotsubo Registry. *J Am Coll Cardiol* 2024; 84(13): 1178-1189. doi: 10.1016/j.jacc.2024.05.076.

6. Lyon, A, Citro, R, Schneider, B. et al. Pathophysiology of Takotsubo syndrome: JACC State-of-the-Art Review. *JACC* 2021; 77(7): 902–921. doi: 10.1016/j.jacc.2020.10.060

7. Becher T, El-Battrawy I, Baumann S, Fastner C, et al. Characteristics and long-term outcome of right ventricular involvement in Takotsubo cardiomyopathy. *International Journal of Cardiology* 2016; 220: 371-375.

8. Yim J. Therapeutic Benefits of Laughter in Mental Health: A Theoretical Review. *Tohoku J Exp Med* 2016; 239(3): 243-249. doi: 10.1620/tjem.239.243. PMID: 27439375.

9. Gupta S, Gupta MM. Takotsubo syndrome. *Indian Heart J* 2018; 70(1): 165-174. doi: 10.1016/j.ihj.2017.09.005. PMID: 29455773; PMCID: PMC5902911.

10. verywell. mind https://www.verywellmind.com (accessed 24 September 2024)

11. Internaional Association for Suicide Prevention https://www.iasp.info/

12. Fuller-Thomson E, Rivière RN, Carrique L, Agbeyaka S. (2020). The Dark Side of ADHD: Factors Associated With Suicide Attempts Among Those With ADHD in a National Representative Canadian Sample. *Archives of Suicide Research* 2020; 26(3): 1122–1140. doi: 10.1080/13811118.2020.1856258

13. Gergel T, Adiukwu F, McInnis M. Suicide and bipolar disorder: opportunities to change the agenda. *Lancet Psychiatry* 2024; 11(10): 781-784. doi: 10.1016/S2215-0366(24)00172-X.

14. Wasserman D, Cheng Q, Jiang GX. Global suicide rates among young people aged 15-19. *World Psychiatry* 2005; 4(2): 114-120. PMID: 16633527; PMCID: PMC1414751.

15. De Leo D, Giannotti AV. Suicide in late life: A viewpoint. *Preventive Medicine* 2021; 152(1): 106735. doi: 10.1016/j.ypmed.2021.106735

16. Browne G. Why suicide rates are dropping around the world. *Wired* 12 May 2023. www.wired.com/story/suicide-prevention-falling-rates/

# Resources

For further information about takotsubo:

Dr Sanjay Gupta's YouTube channel:
www.youtube.com/user/YorkCardiology

Caron Curragh's charity website: www.womensheartbeat.com
Website for information on TTS: www.takotsubo.net
Facebook group:
www.facebook.com/groups/TakotsuboSupport

For help with suicide, these are suicide helplines worldwide:
Algeria:  Emergency: 34342 and 43 Suicide Hotline: 0021 3983 2000 58
Angola: Emergency: 113
Argentina: Emergency: 911 Suicide Hotline: 135
Armenia: Emergency: 911 and 112 Suicide Hotline: (2) 538194
Australia: Emergency: 000 Suicide Hotline: 131114
Austria: Emergency: 112 Telefonseelsorge 24/7: 142
    Rat auf Draht 24/7: 147 (Youth)
Bahamas: Emergency: 911 Suicide Hotline: (2) 322-2763
Bahrain: Emergency: 999
Bangladesh: Emergency: 999
Barbados: Emergency: 911 Suicide Hotline: Samaritan Barbados (246) 4299999
Belgium: Emergency: 112 Suicide Hotline: Stichting Zelfmoordlijn 1813
Bolivia: Emergency: 911 Suicide Hotline: 3911270

Bosnia & Herzegovina: Suicide Hotline: 080 05 03 05
Botswana: Emergency: 911 Suicide Hotline: +2673911270
Brazil: Emergency: 188
Bulgaria: Emergency: 112 Suicide Hotline: 0035 9249 17 223
Burindi: Emergency: 117
Burkina Faso: Emergency: 17
Canada: Emergency: 911 Suicide Hotline: 1 (833) 456 4566
Chad: Emergency: 2251-1237
China: Emergency: 110 Suicide Hotline: 800-810-1117
Colombia: 24/7 Helpline in Barranquilla: 1(00 57 5) 372 27 27 24/7 Hotline Bogota: (57-1) 323 24 25
Congo: Emergency: 117
Costa Rica: Emergency: 911 Suicide Hotline: 506-253-5439
Croatia: Emergency: 112
Cyprus: Emergency: 112 Suicide Hotline: 8000 7773
Czech Republic: Emergency: 112
Denmark: Emergency: 112 Suicide Hotline: 4570201201
Ecuador: Emergency: 911
Egypt: Emergency: 122 Suicide Hotline: 131114
El Salvador: Emergency: 911 Suicide Hotline: 126
Equatorial Guinea: Emergency: 114
Estonia: Emergency: 112 Suicide Hotline: 3726558088; in Russian 3726555688
Ethiopia: Emergency: 911
Finland: Emergency: 112 Suicide Hotline: 010 195 202
France: Emergency: 112 Suicide Hotline: 0145394000
Germany: Emergency: 112 Suicide Hotline: 0800 111 0 111
Ghana: Emergency: 999 Suicide Hotline: 2332 444 71279
Greece: Emergency: 1018
Guatemala: Emergency: 110 Suicide Hotline: 5392-5953
Guinea: Emergency: 117
Guinea Bissau: Emergency: 117
Guyana: Emergency: 999 Suicide Hotline: 223-0001
Holland: Suicide Hotline: 09000767
Hong Kong: Emergency: 999 Suicide Hotline: 852 2382 0000
Hungary: Emergency: 112 Suicide Hotline: 116123
India: Emergency: 112 Suicide Hotline: 8888817666
Indonesia: Emergency: 112 Suicide Hotline: 1-800-273-8255
Iran: Emergency: 110 Suicide Hotline: 1480
Ireland: Emergency: 116123 Suicide Hotline: +4408457909090
Israel: Emergency: 100 Suicide Hotline: 1201

Resources

Italy: Emergency: 112 Suicide Hotline: 800860022
Jamaica: Suicide Hotline: 1-888-429-KARE (5273)
Japan: Emergency: 110 Suicide Hotline: 810352869090
Jordan: Emergency: 911 Suicide Hotline: 110
Kenya: Emergency: 999 Suicide Hotline: 722178177
Kuwait: Emergency: 112 Suicide Hotline: 94069304
Latvia: Emergency: 113 Suicide Hotline: 371 67222922
Lebanon: Suicide Hotline: 1564
Liberia: Emergency: 911 Suicide Hotline: 6534308
Luxembourg: Emergency: 112 Suicide Hotline: 352 45 45 45
Madagascar: Emergency: 117
Malaysia: Emergency: 999 Suicide Hotline: (06) 2842500
Mali: Emergency: 8000-1115
Malta: Suicide Hotline: 179
Mauritius: Emergency: 112 Suicide Hotline: +230 800 93 93
Mexico: Emergency: 911 Suicide Hotline: 5255102550
Netherlands: Emergency: 112 Suicide Hotline: 900 0113
New Zealand: Emergency: 111 Suicide Hotline: 1737
Niger: Emergency: 112
Nigeria: Suicide Hotline: 234 8092106493
Norway: Emergency: 112 Suicide Hotline: +4781533300
Pakistan: Emergency: 115
Philippines: Emergency: 911 Suicide Hotline: 028969191
Poland: Emergency: 112 Suicide Hotline: 5270000
Portugal: Emergency: 112 Suicide Hotline: 21 854 07 40 and 8 96 898 21 50
Qatar: Emergency: 999
Romania: Emergency: 112 Suicide Hotline: 0800 801200
Russia: Emergency: 112 Suicide Hotline: 0078202577577
Saint Vincent and the Grenadines: Suicide Hotline: 9784 456 1044
São Tomé and Príncipe: Suicide Hotline: (239) 222-12-22 ext. 123
Saudi Arabia: Emergency: 112
Serbia: Suicide Hotline: (+381) 21-6623-393
Senegal: Emergency: 17
Singapore: Emergency: 999 Suicide Hotline: 1 800 2214444
Spain: Emergency: 112 Suicide Hotline: 914590050
South Africa: Emergency: 10111 Suicide Hotline: 0514445691
South Korea: Emergency: 112 Suicide Hotline: (02) 7158600
Sri Lanka: Suicide Hotline: 011 057 2222662
Sudan: Suicide Hotline: (249) 11-555-253
Sweden: Emergency: 112 Suicide Hotline: 46317112400
Switzerland: Emergency: 112 Suicide Hotline: 143

Tanzania: Emergency: 112
Thailand: Suicide Hotline: (02) 713-6793
Tonga: Suicide Hotline: 23000
Trinidad and Tobago: Suicide Hotline: (868) 645 2800
Tunisia: Emergency: 197
Turkey: Emergency: 112
Uganda: Emergency: 112 Suicide Hotline: 0800 21 21 21
United Arab Emirates: Suicide Hotline: 800 46342
United Kingdom: Emergency: 999 Suicide Hotline: 0800 689 5652 Samaritans 116123
United States: Emergency: 911 Suicide Hotline: 988
Zambia: Emergency: 999 Suicide Hotline: +260960264040
Zimbabwe: Emergency: 999 Suicide Hotline: 080 1

# Index

**A**
AA meetings, 31, 32
abdominal breathing, 160
abdominal pain, 154
ACE inhibitors, 97
ADHD, suicide risk factor, 213, 214
adrenaline, 82, 111
    dental treatment and, 164, 167
adrenaline-inducing sports/
    situations, 111, 156, 158
age
    suicide rates by, 215
    takotsubo syndrome and, 112
air ambulance, 158
alcohol consumption, takotsubo
    events due to, 106
Alexandra's story, 141–143
Alex's story, 127–129
anger, 9
    at A&E staff, 155
    grief stage, 44
    Juliet's *see under* Sullivan,
        Juliet
    in personal stories, 129, 139,
        155, 156
angina, 153, 162, 163

angiogram, 62, 94, 115
    description, 115
    for Juliet Sullivan, 62
    TTS diagnosis, 62, 94
Anita's story, 135–137
anti-histamines, 101
anxiety, 135
    after takotsubo event, 70, 84,
        144
    managing, 85, 86, 91, 118, 119,
        155
    takotsubo trigger, 122
apical ballooning syndrome, xiii
    *see also* takotsubo (TTS)
        cardiomyopathy
arm pain, 146
arrhythmia, 116
asthma, 105–106
atrial fibrillation (AF, Afib), 116
atrium (atria), 116
author's personal story *see*
    Sullivan, Juliet

**B**
Barbara's story, 137–141
baths, benefits, 86

Abbreviations: TTS – takotsubo/takotsubo cardiomyopathy
Note: Recipes are all grouped under 'recipes'.

beta-blocker, in personal stories, 144, 145, 157, 159, 166
'bikini medicine' model, ix
bipolar disorder, suicide risk, 214
bisoprolol, 122
blood pressure
   elevated, 82, 125
      in personal stories, 123, 125, 133, 141, 142, 149, 167
   low, in personal stories, 136, 155, 166
   monitoring, after takotsubo event, 120, 126
blood test, for troponin see troponin
bradycardia, 116, 160
breathing
   abdominal, 160
   deep, 86–87
breathlessness/breathing difficulty
   after recovery from TTS, 121, 138, 148, 157, 159, 167
   diagnosis of takotsubo without, 113
   onset of TTS, stories, 117, 125, 128, 130, 147, 149, 150, 161, 163
'broken heart'
   dying from, 79, 147
   symptoms, 61
'broken heart syndrome,' xiii, xiv, 61, 79, 80, 82
   opinions on label/name, xiii–xiv, 109
   see also takotsubo (TTS) cardiomyopathy
butterfly, sign, 49

## C

caffeine, 87
cardiac ablation, viii
cardiac arrest, 161
   see also heart attack
cardiac catheterisation see angiogram
cardiologist, knowledgeable, importance of finding, viii, 123, 124, 142
cardiomyopathy
   definition, 97, 116
   takotsubo see takotsubo (TTS) cardiomyopathy
Carmel's story, 164–167
Carol's story, 146–148
cataplexy, 106
catecholamines, 82
Catherine's story, 152–156
catheterisation, heart see angiogram
charity, Women's Heartbeat, ix
chest, compression feeling, 58
chest pain, 107–108
   during dental treatment, 120
   diagnosis of takotsubo without, 113
   investigations, 94–95
   in personal stories, vii, 120, 121, 125, 130, 136, 138, 143, 149, 150, 152, 153, 156–157, 158, 159, 163, 165
chest x-ray, 59, 143
chip pan fire, 17–18
cholesterol, raised, 164
Claire's story, 121–124
clinical trials, on takotsubo, 71–72, 104
clopidogrel, 122
cognitive behavioural therapy (CBT), 90, 107
cold-water swimming, 111
coma, 161
confounding bias, 108
consciousness, loss of, 117, 128
coronary arteries, normal in takotsubo, 82
counselling, 90–91
   in personal stories, 126, 127, 145
COVID, 101, 124, 130, 132, 137

# Index

COVID-19 vaccine, 164, 166
Curragh, Caron
    clinical paper on TTS, viii–ix
    takotsubo event, vii–viii
    website, viii, 221
cyclic sighing, 86
cycling, 137, 167

## D

David's story, 119–121
Dawson, Professor Dana, 71, 90, 98, 100
    interview with, ix, 104–114
    qualifications, 104
    research on TTS, 104–105
deaths due to takotsubo, 72, 95, 109
defibrillating vest, 150–151
defibrillator, implanted, 161–162
dehydration, 96
dental treatment, 120, 164, 167
depression, 84
    Juliet's mother's, 36
    post-takotsubo, 113–114
    situational, suicidal ideation, 214
    suicide risk factor, 214
detachment, 55, 58
diagnosis of takotsubo, vii–viii, 94
    heart attack vs, 94–95
    Juliet Sullivan's, 57, 58, 67
    misdiagnosis, 108
    tests, 62, 94–95
    without chest pain/breathing difficulty, 113
    *see also* angiogram; troponin
diet
    changes, recovery from TTS, 91–92
    healthy, 61, 103–104, 135, 171
    role in takotsubo syndrome, 91, 103–104, 106
    *see also* recipes
dietary fibre, 91
dietary supplements, natural, 101–102
diltiazem, 149
discharge from hospital, 64, 100, 111
diuretics, 97
dopamine, 82, 87
dread, sense of, 58, 117
driving, stress related to, 65–66
dry drowning, 117–118
'dying of a broken heart', 79, 147

## E

ECG (electrocardiogram), 95, 113
    Juliet Sullivan's, 59, 60
    in personal stories, 136, 138, 143, 149, 153, 165
echocardiogram, 95, 97, 115–116
    in personal stories, 125, 131, 139, 142, 157, 165
education/training of doctors, 69, 103
ejection fraction (EF), 62, 81–82, 116
    definition/description, 62, 81, 116
    low, in TTS, 62, 81–82, 116, 128
    Juliet Sullivan's, 62
    personal stories, 118, 128, 144, 150, 151, 153
    normal level, 62, 81, 116
electric shock treatment, 26
Elinor's story, 130–132
Emergency Room (ER), cardiac symptoms of TTS being ignored, 150, 151
emotion(s), 3, 131
    hiding, 3, 63, 131
    releasing, 86, 89, 132

---

Abbreviations: TTS – takotsubo/takotsubo cardiomyopathy
Note: Recipes are all grouped under 'recipes'.

emotional pain/stress, 34, 47, 73, 80
    catecholamine release, 82
    in personal stories, 120, 128, 131, 144, 155, 161
    *see also* stress
endorphins, 114
epinephrine *see* adrenaline
Epsom salt bath, 86
exercise, 84
    concerns over, after takotsubo event, 140
    high intensity interval training (HIIT), 114, 138
    moderate, after takotsubo event, 167
    recovery of heart and brain, 84, 107
exhaustion *see* fatigue; tiredness/exhaustion
eye movement desensitisation and reprocessing therapy (EMDR), 145

**F**
Facebook group for takotsubo patients, viii, 83–84, 145, 159, 167
fatigue, after takotsubo event, 108
    in personal stories, 122, 140, 148, 153, 157–158, 159, 166, 167
    *see also* tiredness/exhaustion
fears, after takotsubo event
    Juliet Sullivan's, 17, 26, 69, 70, 73, 74, 84–85
    in personal stories, 118, 125, 129, 144, 145, 148
Fifi (piece of wood), 20–21
fight-or-flight response, 100, 160
flying and travel after takotsubo event
    Juliet Sullivan's, 69
    in personal stories, 162, 163, 164
forgiveness, 53
friends
    Juliet's *see* Sullivan, Juliet
    reaching out/connecting with, 88
funerals, 114, 135
    Juliet's mother's, 42, 43

**G**
gadolinium, 95
genetic vulnerability, 99, 100, 101
gigs, 6, 63
GPs, takotsubo knowledge and training, 103
grains, in diet, 91, 92
grief, 8, 10, 40
    for lost health, stories, 139
    for Margaret (Juliet's mother), 39, 40, 44, 63, 73–74
    as process, 49, 63–64
    stages of, 44
    suppressing, adverse effects of, 64
    for Susan, 8, 10, 62–63
GTN (glyceryl trinitrate) spray, 120, 125, 162, 163
guided meditation, 87
Gupta, Dr Sanjay
    interview with, ix, 93–103
    YouTube channel, 221

**H**
hatha yoga, 85
heart
    anatomy, 81, 82
    blood flow through, 81, 82, 116
    damage in takotsubo, 94, 155
    enlargement (left ventricle), 66, 81, 82, 96–97, 157, 165
    functional status, assessment, 98
    health of, check-up after takotsubo, 64, 66–67
    inflammatory cells in, 109

## Index

movements, 97–98
normal, 82
normalisation of function after TTS, 97–98
rate *see* heart rate
rhythm, abnormal, 116
scarring, 95, 96
shape, in takotsubo, 81, 82, 96, 97, 136
stabbing pain, 107–108
subtle abnormalities after takotsubo, 98, 100
as three-dimensional structure, 97–98
weak, after takotsubo event, 81, 96, 98, 100
weakness, assessment, 97
heart attack, 93–94, 95–96
   diagnostic tests, 94–95, 113
   heart muscle damage, 94, 95
   Juliet's initial diagnosis, 60, 61, 62, 65, 67
   NSTEMI, 117, 151
   personal stories, 118, 122, 123–124, 125, 127, 130, 133, 134, 138, 141, 143, 147, 153, 154, 157
   in post-menopausal women, 112
   risk factors, 105
   silent, 138, 139
   takotsubo caused by, 113
   takotsubo causing, 113
   takotsubo diagnosis vs, 94–95
   takotsubo differences, 93–94
   tests, 94–95
   takotsubo misdiagnosis as, 108
   troponin level, 95, 115
heartbeat, 116

heart 'cath' (catheterisation) *see* angiogram
heart failure, vii, viii, 61, 116, 125
'heart failure patient', 142
heart-healthy recipes *see* recipes, heart-healthy
heart rate
   fast (tachycardia), 116
   normal, 116
   in personal stories, 130, 133, 138, 149, 151, 155
   slow (bradycardia), 116, 160
heart rehab, 67
heart rhythm, abnormal, 116
Heather's story, 162–164
high intensity interval training (HIIT), 114, 138
histamine, 100
hobbies, 89–90
HRT (hormone replacement therapy), 112

**I**
inflammatory cells, in heart, 109
inflammatory reaction, 109
information booklets, on takotsubo, 68
information sources, on takotsubo, 221
inquest into Juliet's mother's death, 51–53
InterTAK study, 71–72
isolation, desire for, 88

**J**
jar of joy, 42
journal, keeping a, 89
Juliet's story, 148–152
Juliet Sullivan's story *see* Sullivan, Juliet

Abbreviations: TTS – takotsubo/takotsubo cardiomyopathy
Note: Recipes are all grouped under 'recipes'.

**K**
Karen (Juliet's sister), xi, 13, 14, 19, 20
  burns and hospital visit, 17–18
  mother's depression and need of help, 36, 37
  mother's inquest, 51, 52, 53
  visits to mother in psychiatric hospital, 25
Kerri (Juliet's daughter), 7, 26–27, 54
  after Juliet's diagnosis, 62
  response when Juliet taken ill, 58
  wedding, 7, 44–45
kidneys, in takotsubo syndrome, 96, 97
knowledge about takotsubo syndrome, 84, 103
  lack of, viii, xiv, 68, 73, 98, 108, 113, 162

**L**
laughing yoga, 88
laughter, xv, 62, 87–88
  cataplexy, 106
Lee (Juliet's husband), 5, 6, 10, 27, 41, 47
  after Juliet's mother's suicide, 49, 53, 54
  support for Juliet after takotsubo, 56, 62
  Susan's death, 7
Lee Ann's story, 143–146
left ventricle, 81
  blood flow through, 82, 116
  enlarged in takotsubo syndrome, 66, 81, 82, 96–97, 157, 165
left ventricular ejection fraction, 81–82
  *see also* ejection fraction (EF)
legumes, in diet, 92
Liam (Juliet's son), 27, 47, 48
  after Juliet's diagnosis, 62

gig, 63
lifestyle, 113
  changes after takotsubo, in stories, 140, 160
  changes for recovery, 91–92
  healthy, 91–92, 103–104
Linda's story, 156–160
Lipton, Bruce H, 100
listening to patients, 98
longevity, supplements and, 102
Lori's story, 133–135

**M**
magnetic resonance imaging (MRI), 95
Margaret (Juliet's mother)
  absences from home during Juliet's childhood, 18, 23
  alcoholism, 11, 24, 31, 32
  anger, 49
  butterfly, sign from, 49
  death *see suicide* (below)
  depression, 36–37
  funeral, 42–43
  GP's care of, 52–53
  inquest into death, 51–53
  mental illness, 11, 24, 25
  'octopus' (safe word), 33, 57
  overdose and suicide attempts, 10, 11, 15, 23–27, 36
  electric shock treatment (ECT), 26
  first suicide attempt, 11, 15, 23–24
  recording about her life, 55
  relationship with Juliet, 9–10, 11, 15, 18, 19, 21, 24, 27, 55
  Canadian visit, 31, 32–33
  cutting off contact, 29–30
  as villain of Juliet's childhood, 19, 21
  relationship with other people, 30, 31–32, 42, 48
  residential care home, 37

## Index

sense of entitlement, 31
sight problems, 11, 30, 32
suicide, 35–38, 49
   date, 35, 63
   Juliet's reaction, 35–36, 39–40, 47–48, 49, 74
   visit to Canada, 29–34
      depression after, 36–37
      invitation from Juliet, 29, 30
      Juliet's memories of visit, 30–34, 48
      reassurance and end of visit, 34
   visit to clairvoyant, 37–38
Marian's story, 124–127
medications in takotsubo, 97
   anti-histamines, 101
   effectiveness, assessment, 108
   in personal stories, 120–121, 123, 126, 144, 157, 163, 166
   second episode prevention and, 99, 101
meditation, 87, 127
'memory pain', heart, 107–108
men
   suicide statistics, 213–214
   takotsubo in, 72, 80, 106, 110
menopause
   information on, 92
   post-menopause and takotsubo, 68, 80, 112
mental health conditions, 113–114
mental wellbeing rehabilitation, 107
metoprolol, 149
Mia (Juliet's friend), xi, 8–9, 10, 52, 53
mind–body connection, 72, 74, 105–106, 131, 145

morphine, 158, 160
MRI in takotsubo, 95
music, 89
myocardial infarction *see* heart attack

**N**
natural supplements, 101–102
nausea and vomiting, 117–118, 128, 133, 146, 161, 163, 165
Neild, Kerri, 90
NSTEMI (non-ST-elevation myocardial infarction), 117, 151
Nutini, Paolo, 6, 63

**O**
'octopus' (as safe word), 33, 57
octopus-trap (takotsubo), xiii, xv, 82
oxytocin, 75

**P**
pacemaker, 160
pain
   abdominal, 154
   chest *see* chest pain
   extreme, in story of takotsubo event, 154–155
   shoulder, 128, 130, 141, 146
   stabbing, in heart, 107–108
palpitations, 108
panic attack, 56, 58, 60, 85
Paolo Nutini gig, 6, 63
personal stories
   of author *see* Sullivan, Juliet
   of Caron Curragh, vii–viii
   of TTS patients *see* stories of takotsubo
pesticides, suicide and, 216

Abbreviations: TTS – takotsubo/takotsubo cardiomyopathy
Note: Recipes are all grouped under 'recipes'.

physical exercise *see* exercise
physical illness, as trigger for takotsubo, 105–106
poltergeist, 16
positive, staying, 119
post-menopausal women, takotsubo affecting, 68, 80, 112, 157
psychosomatic interaction, 105, 106
'punch-drunk state' of heart muscle, 94

**Q**
quality of life, 102

**R**
recipes, heart-healthy, 171–206
  breakfast, 172–176
    berry smoothie, 176
    chia seed pudding with fruit, 173
    healthy burrito wrap, 175
    other suggestions, 176
    protein-packed pancakes, 174
    tofu scramble with spinach, 172
    wholegrain toast with peanut butter and banana-cinnamon, 173
  desserts, 200–206
    avocado chocolate pudding, 202
    baked apples, 203
    blueberry yogurt clusters, 202
    dark chocolate cashew clusters, 204
    fruit skewers, 206
    healthy chocolate mousse, 201
    healthy fudge brownies, 205
    watermelon fruit pizza, 200
  dinner, 188–199
    chickpea chicken dinner bowl, 196–197
    chickpea meatballs with spaghetti, 198–199
    easy veggie chilli, 188
    grilled chicken barley bowl, 190
    healthy baked salmon, 195
    healthy fish tacos, 192–194
    kale, ginger and sweet potato stew with lentils and coconut milk, 191–192
    sheet-pan cashew chicken, 189
  lunch, 177–187
    baked sweet potatoes and fillings, 187
    chicken and cucumber lettuce wraps with peanut sauce, 186–187
    chickpea salad, 177
    chopped cobb salad with chicken, 182
    creamy sweet potato soup, 184–185
    curry lentil soup, 179–180
    honey mustard vinaigrette, 184
    mason-jar power salad with chickpeas and tuna, 183
    Mediterranean tuna salad, 178
    Mexican-style baked sweet potatoes, 180–181
    other suggestions, 187
    wholegrain sandwiches and fillings, 187
    wholegrain wraps and fillings, 187
  snacks, 207–211
    carrot fries, 209
    choccie blueberries, 208
    crispy smashed Brussels

sprouts, 210
easy garlicky kale, 207
high-protein flaxseed
  bread, 210–211
other suggestions, 211
recovery after takotsubo event,
  83–92
  advice for, 110
  discharge from hospital/care,
    64, 100, 111
  pacing and time required for,
    110
  in personal stories, 118–119,
    120–121, 123, 125–126, 129,
    134–135, 136, 151–152, 158,
    159, 160, 162, 164, 167
  problems ongoing after six
    months, viii, 98, 110, 111,
    118–119
  time required for, 69–70, 72,
    96, 110
recovery after takotsubo event,
  suggestions for, 83–92, 110
  abdominal breathing, 160
  adequate sleep, 88–89
  avoiding unhealthy habits, 87
  breath work/deep breathing,
    86–87
  connecting with other people,
    88
  counselling, 90–91
  cyclic sighing, 86
  dietary changes, 91–92, 171
  Epsom salt bath, 86
  exercise, 84, 107
  hobby, taking up, 89–90
  keeping a journal, 89
  laughter, 87–88
  lifestyle changes, 91–92
  making yourself a priority, 88
  meditation, 87

from personal stories, 127,
  136–137, 140–141, 143, 145,
  146, 160
research, 83–84
swimming, 85
walking, 84–85
yoga, 85
yoga nidra, 86
recurrence of takotsubo event, x,
  106–107
  avoidance, 99, 101
  causes/stressors, x, 112
  likelihood of second event,
    106–107
  in personal stories, x, 124, 153,
    158, 159–160
refusal to acknowledge serious
  problem, 58, 59
registry data, 71–72, 108
research on takotsubo, 68,
  104–105
  clinical trial/study, 71–72, 104
  funding, 110
  men's vs women's heart
    health, ix–x
  by patients, 83–84
  scientific papers, viii–ix, 71–72
  in women, 110
right ventricle, 81

S
Sabine's story, 161–162
Sato, Dr Hikaru, xv
scientific papers, viii–ix, 71–72
Scottish Takotsubo Registry, 107
screening for takotsubo
  syndrome, 99
*The Secret* (Rhonda Byrne), 48,
  49
self-education, x, 92, 146
Shannon (Juliet's friend), 48

Abbreviations: TTS – takotsubo/takotsubo cardiomyopathy
Note: Recipes are all grouped under 'recipes'.

shortness of breath *see*
    breathlessness/breathing
    difficulty
shoulder pain, 128, 130, 141, 146
sleep
    difficulties, 88, 138, 156
    duration, requirements, 148,
        163
    getting enough and
        improving, 86, 88–89
sleep aids, 86
socialising, 88
somatic therapy, 74, 75, 90–91
    relational, 90–91
    touch your heart technique, 75
sports, adrenaline-inducing, 111
statins, 164
stories of takotsubo, xiv, 115–167
    Alexandra's, 141–143
    Alex's, 127–129
    Anita's, 135–137
    Barbara's, 137–141
    Carmel's, 164–167
    Carol's, 146–148
    Catherine's, 152–156
    Claire's, 121–124
    Curragh, Caron's, vii–viii
    David's, 119–121
    Elinor's, 130–132
    Heather's, 162–164
    Juliet's, 148–152
    Lee Ann's, 143–146
    Linda's, 156–160
    Lori's, 133–135
    Marian's, 124–127
    Sabine's, 161–162
    Sullivan, Juliet's *see* Sullivan,
        Juliet
    Valerie's, 117–119
stress, 97
    author's story, 3, 4, 69, 70, 72
    avoidance, 73, 114
    catecholamines released, 82
    chronic, histamine and, 100
    cumulative, ix

life without, 64, 65–70
management, 3, 83
reduction techniques, 75, 83,
    85, 86–87, 87–88, 89, 126
as takotsubo trigger, 80, 83, 97,
    105, 144
    in personal stories, 117,
        122, 125, 131–132, 161,
        162–163
stress hormones, 80
stress-induced cardiomyopathy,
    97
suicidal ideation, 43, 213
    ADHD as risk factor, 213, 214
    help for and talking about,
        216–217
    helplines, 216, 221–224
    Juliet's mother's, 9–10
suicide, 54, 213–217
    ADHD link, 213, 214
    age relationship, 215
    attempted, 214
    bipolar disorder link, 214
    downward trend, 215–216
    helplines, 216, 221–224
    by Margaret *see* Margaret
        (Juliet's mother)
    method/means of, 216
    rates by country, 215, 216
    risk factors, 214
    statistics, 213–214
suicide bereavement support
    group, 54–55
Sullivan, Juliet, 3–76
    anger with mother, 9, 10, 21,
        24, 43, 44
    after her death, 41, 49, 55
    at funeral, 41, 42–43
    belief in attracting what is
        wanted, 48, 49
    birth, 15
    business, 69
    butterfly sign, 49
    in Canada (expat), 3, 5, 6–7, 27
        return after mother's

funeral, 47
childhood (troubled), 13–21
chip pan fire, and reaction to, 17–18
daily achievements, 53–54
damage from mother's illness, 11
daughter *see* Kerri (Juliet's daughter)
dog (Hallie) and ball, 48
exhaustion, 30, 33–34
family home, 16
father
    arrangement to see, 18–19
    living with, 25–26
    relationship with, 19, 20
father's death, 9
fears, feelings of, 17, 26, 69, 70, 73, 74, 84–85
feelings for mother, 9–10, 27, 29, 30, 32–33, 55
    *see also* Margaret (Juliet's mother)
feeling unwell at support group, 55–56
Fifi (wood), 20–21
friends, 27, 29
    Mia, xi, 8–9, 10, 52, 53
    Shannon, 48
    Susan and her death, 7–8, 10, 29, 32, 34, 62–63
grief
    over mother's death, 39, 40, 44, 63, 73–74
    over Susan's death, 8, 10, 62–63
guilt over mother, 10, 27, 30, 33, 34, 43
healthy lifestyle, 61
heart break, and regret, 50, 51, 55–56, 61–62, 75

husband (Lee) *see* Lee (Juliet's husband)
inquest into mother's death, 51–53
insulting mother, 41
laughter, default reaction, 62
lifestyle, 3, 6
life without stress, 64, 65–70
memories of childhood, 13, 16, 20, 21
memories of mother's visit to Canada, 48
mother's suicide
    reaction to, 35–36, 39–40, 47–48, 49, 74
    return to England after, 40–42
    as mother to Kerri and Liam, 6, 7
music festival, 5, 7
'octopus' (safe word), 33, 57
panic attacks, 56, 58, 60, 85
parents' divorce, 11, 13–14, 15, 16
parents' marriage, 15
personal hygiene, 15–16
personality, 43
relationship with mother *see* under Margaret (Juliet's mother)
running away (Finland, Spain, Canada), 26, 27
sister *see* Karen (Juliet's sister)
somatic therapy, 74, 75, 90
son (Liam) *see* Liam (Juliet's son)
stress/stressful events, 3, 4, 69, 70, 72
    at suicide bereavement support group, 54–55
takotsubo event, ix

Abbreviations: TTS – takotsubo/takotsubo cardiomyopathy
Note: Recipes are all grouped under 'recipes'.

aftermath, 71–76
background to, 3–4, 5–11, 62–64
changing thoughts after, 74, 75
concerns/feelings after, 66, 69, 70, 72, 73, 84
diagnosis, 57, 58, 62, 67
diagnosis, feelings about, 61–62
discharge, 64
Emergency department, 59, 60
examination and history, 59, 60–61
fears after, 69, 70, 73, 74, 84–85
flying/travel after, 69
fragility after, 69, 70, 73
heart attack diagnosis, 60, 61, 62
heart health after, 64, 66–67, 73
life after, 69–70, 73, 84
medication, 66, 67
mental health recovery after, 72, 73
recovery and lifestyle after, 61, 67, 69, 73
recovery period duration, 69–70, 72
stress after, and responses, 69, 70, 72
symptoms, 58
tiredness/exhaustion after, 66, 69, 72
walking after, 84–85
visits to mother in psychiatric hospital, 25
writing (books), 54
yoga, 85–86
support groups, viii, 143, 145, 151–152, 159
Facebook group, viii, 83–84, 145, 159, 167

supraventricular tachycardia (SVT), 116–117
in personal stories, 149, 151
Susan's (Juliet's friend), death, 7–8, 10, 29, 32, 34, 62–63
swimming, 85, 117, 163
cold-water, 111
symptoms of takotsubo event, 82
cardiac symptoms ignored, 150, 151
chest pain *see* chest pain
duration, 98, 107–108
nausea/vomiting, 117–118, 128, 133, 146, 161, 163, 165
shoulder pain, 128, 130, 141, 146

**T**

tachycardia, 116
takotsubo (octopus-trap), xiii, xv, 82
takotsubo (TTS) cardiomyopathy, xiii, xiv, 61, 79–81
age spectrum, 112
anxiety and fragility after event, 70
care limited for, 68–69
catecholamines and, 82
causes/triggers, vii, xiv, 80, 97, 105–106, 112, 122, 160
physical triggers, increase in, 72
stress *see* stress
cause unknown, 80–81, 160
complications, 107, 151–152
damage reversible, 61–62, 94
deaths due to, 72, 95, 109
depression after, 113–114
description/definition, 79–81
diagnosis *see* diagnosis of takotsubo
expert opinions, 93–114
Dawson, Dana, 104–114
Gupta, Sanjay, 93–103
genetic vulnerability, 99, 100, 101

GP awareness about, 103
heart attack causing/after, 113
heart attack differences, 93–94
immediate hospital attendance, 96, 107
lack of knowledge about, viii, xiv, 68, 73, 98, 108, 113, 162
left ventricle in, 66, 81, 82, 96–97, 157, 165
medications for *see* medications in takotsubo
in men, 72, 80, 106, 110
misconception as trivial condition, viii, x, xiii
misdiagnosis, 108
newly diagnosed, advice for, 110
origin of name, xiii, xv, 82
post-menopausal women, 68, 80, 112, 157
post-mortem examinations (autopsies), 96, 109
prevalence, 93
prevention, 64
'punch-drunk state' of heart muscle, 94
recovery *see* recovery after takotsubo event
recurrence *see* recurrence of takotsubo event
research *see* research
reversible and recovery, 61–62, 94
risk factors, 80
screening, 99
second event *see* recurrence of takotsubo event
specialists on, 67–68
stories *see* stories of takotsubo
subtle heart abnormalities after, 98

symptoms *see* symptoms of takotsubo
treatment, 83, 108
unrecognised, and deaths due to, 79
'why me?' question, 105–106
in women, research and, 110
tiredness/exhaustion after takotsubo, 98, 108
duration, 108
Juliet Sullivan's, 72
in personal stories, 119, 121, 122, 125, 135, 136, 138, 140, 142, 144, 158
*see also* fatigue
touch your heart technique, 75
travel *see* flying and travel after takotsubo event
troponin, 95, 113, 115
description, 115
in personal stories, 60, 118, 124, 134, 136, 139, 141, 143, 150, 153, 157, 165
return to normal after attack, 115, 154
significance, 95, 154
TTS (*or* TS) *see* takotsubo (TTS) cardiomyopathy
TTS support group *see* support groups

**U**
unhealthy habits, 87

**V**
vaccines, takotsubo link, 112
Valerie's story, 117–119
vegetables, 91
ventricles, enlargement, 66, 81, 82, 96–97, 157, 165
vibration sensation, 141

Abbreviations: TTS – takotsubo/takotsubo cardiomyopathy
Note: Recipes are all grouped under 'recipes'.

vitamin C, 102
volunteering, 88
vomiting (and nausea), 117–118, 128, 133, 146, 161, 163, 165

**W**
walking, after takotsubo event, 84–85
weakness, 98
website, for TTS, viii
wedding, Kerri's (Juliet's daughter), 7, 44–45
wine, 56, 61, 73, 87
women
    post-menopausal, takotsubo in, 68, 80, 112, 157
    as second-class citizens for heart health, ix, xi
    suicide statistics, 213–214
Women's Heartbeat, ix

**Y**
yoga, 3, 35, 85
    laughing, 88
yoga nidra, 86
yourself, making a priority, 88

**Z**
ziplining, 111

# Also from Hammersmith Books...

## The Getting of Resilience from the Inside Out

### By Sally Baker

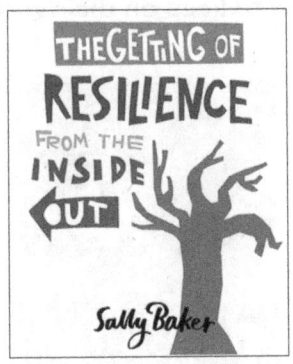

To combat physical nasties we need a strong immune system. To combat negative life events we need resilience. Here award-winning therapist Sally Baker gives us a practical guide to developing a wider understanding of resilience and to fostering it so that we have the essential perseverance and drive to emerge successfully when confronted with life's inevitable and often unexpected challenges. Sally explores some of the key family dynamics that can result in unhelpful ways of thinking about oneself which may undermine the natural development of resilience and in its place impose a cycle of self-sabotaging behaviour. Coping strategies such as heightened anxiety, non-confrontational behaviour, people-pleasing habits, along with 'adult failure to thrive', are just a few of the learnt strategies often originally forged out of powerlessness in response to less than ideal early life experiences. These strategies, however, can be re-assessed and the misplaced guilt, shame and self-blame that have affixed these behaviours, often for many years, can be resolved and released, making way for the getting of resilience from the inside out.

# Also from the author of What Becomes of the Broken-hearted?...

## The Gallstone-friendly Diet (Second Edition)
### Everything you never wanted to know about gallstones (and hot to keep on their good side)

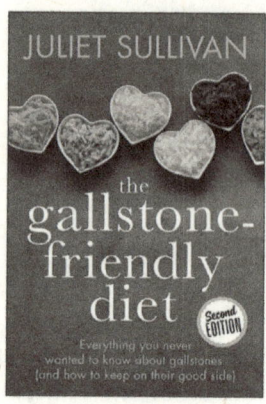

Every year in the UK around 66,000 people have their gallbladder removed because of gallstones. The figure for Ireland is over 20,000. This number has been increasing year on year into a virtual epidemic, almost certainly related to contemporary high sugar/fructose diets. But it is fats that bring on gallstone symptoms – 'gallbladder colic', said to be one of the most acutely painful experiences we can have.

While seeking treatment for gallstones, the only way to avoid this pain is to follow a no-fat or very low-fat diet so that the gallbladder is not stimulated into action. But how to change the habits of a life time? Juliet Sullivan has been on that journey and, with her usual candour and wit, shares what she has learned along the way (now in an expanded second edition), including what worked for her and the recipes she developed that saw her through to surgery and beyond.

With star ratings for fat levels, her guidance is quick and easy to follow and provides low-fat alternatives for family favourites – from a roast dinner to spag bol – so sufferers can eat with family and friends and not feel excluded on account of their medical problem.